CAREGIVING

CAREGIVING

Eldercare Made Clear and Simple

Cindy Laverty

CLW
PUBLISHING

CLW Publishing
4570 Van Nuys Blvd., Suite 184
Van Nuys, California 91403
Phone: 818-623-3011
Fax: 818-302-1688

Author photo on cover by Starla Fortunato

PRINTED IN THE UNITED STATES OF AMERICA

ISBN: 978-0-9827765-0-6

Dedication

This book is dedicated to all caregivers who search for ways to make life as seamless as possible for the elderly and who create peaceful, harmonious solutions in another human being's life.

I could not have survived without my family who always offered support, and gave me numerous "free passes" for bad behavior. I thank them for simply putting up with me while I was going through the process. The support and encouragement they gave me meant more than they will ever know.

And to Robert, who gave me the courage and strength to forge into areas I knew nothing about, I will always treasure this precious time in my life. Thank you, pal.

Contents

A Word From Cindy

There are thousands of books that address the subject of caregiving, and I have read a good number of them. I list some of the most valuable at the end of this manual. I wanted to create a useful guide that was based on my personal experiences and I wanted this information to be simple and concise because, if you are a caregiver or think you will become one, the last thing you want to do at the end of the day is read a book on this subject. The truth is that I read most of these books long after the circumstances that provided me with this expertise. I had no time. I needed something functional and I needed help. I needed to escape, and books on caregiving were not the answer for me.

This is a care guide that is designed to be adaptable. Caregiver needs change over time and some sections may seem unnecessary now, but may be helpful in the future.

Please let me know if the ideas and forms work for you, and send me your suggestions. I am always looking for improvements and I welcome your feedback.

Please, email me at: Cindy@thecarecompany.biz.

Cindy Laverty

Introduction

If you are in a position to use this manual, you can take comfort in knowing that you are *not* alone. The subject of caring for our aging population is commonplace in all social circles. Everyone is affected by the need to provide proper care delivered with dignity and respect to our aging population. Few of us know what to do.

Several years ago, I was one of those people literally thrown into a situation I knew nothing about. I was asked by my former father-in-law, Bob, (with whom I had a close relationship) to pay his bills and check on his wife (who suffered from severe arthritis and dementia) while he had open-heart surgery at eighty-three years of age. His reason for having such invasive and risky surgery was so he could see his granddaughter (my daughter) graduate from college and, as he said to me, "Without this operation, I won't make it."

You can imagine the impact of such a statement. I agreed without giving it any further thought, never imagining that I would someday write a manual designed to help others in similar situations who do not know where to get help. I naively thought this promise to help out would be a minor investment of my time. For a number of complicated reasons, I was the only person who was capable of stepping forward to care for Bob and his wife, and I was honored that he trusted me to handle this role. I'm certain that neither of us realized the impact it would have on both of our lives and our relationship.

Even though we shared a close relationship, I was, aware enough to know that, if I were to have control of a checkbook that didn't belong to me, I wanted and needed to have proper legal forms in place. I had to be "bulletproof" or as bulletproof as possible. Bob and I met with his family attorney and, with the signing of a couple of documents and the signature and stamp of a notary, we made the arrangement legal. I still knew nothing about this process and it's a good thing I didn't, because I probably would never have taken it on. This is not meant to scare you, only to point out that you need to be prepared!

The fourteen-hour operation was only the beginning of what became the most fascinating education of my life. I knew nothing of the geriatric world or the needs of those living in it. I learned quickly about hospitals, doctors, nurses, protocols, bureaucracy, insurance forms, Medicare, prescription drugs, and how to manage them. I learned how easy it is to get lost in this system and, consequently, I spent a good portion of the first year learning how to avoid being abused by the system. My learning curve had to be swift and precise. I was fortunate in that I was dealing with wonderful doctors who truly cared about their patient, but they were still doctors with very little extra time. It was quickly evident that chitchat was not going to be a part of this process. I had to ask questions and be clear. Clarity is key to success.

My agreement to pay bills and check on Bob's wife turned very quickly into a full-time obligation. She was suffering from severe dementia and her caregivers were not properly caring for her. The key to keeping her in a peaceful, unagitated state was the proper administration of her mediations, which required special attention. The house was in disrepair.

The staff needed replacement. The new staff needed training. The bills needed attention. Past due bills needed immediate attention. Visits to the hospital were daily; morning and early evening, with emergencies added to the mix. After a few weeks I managed to create a schedule that worked for everyone, with the exception of me.

Then, it happened. The doctors had warned that it might and it did. A stroke. Not a major, life-threatening stroke, but a debilitating stroke, nonetheless. Everything changed and Bob's recovery would be all the more difficult. Suddenly he was off to a new hospital where no one knew him, and everything was unfamiliar. He would have to rehabilitate in a new facility. Depression slowly set in as he worked to improve his functionality, while knowing that the activities he once participated in were no longer a part of his life. After a month of rehab, he returned home.

My responsibility didn't stop here. There were numerous medical issues to deal with: insomnia, depression, seizures, weakness, incontinence, functionality, balance, and the overall day-to-day challenges that the elderly experience when life begins to take its toll on the body.

Clearly, my role was not going to be temporary. If you had told me many years ago that I'd be a caregiver for my ex-father-in-law, I would have thought you were crazy. But this became my life. I didn't have time to think about the consequences of this change for me; I had work to do and I wasn't going to let him down. I was on call 24/7, 365 days a year. I visited him daily. Sometimes we had beautiful visits with laughter and remembrances, and then there were those other days when he was just mad at the world and I received the brunt of his anger (does any of this sound familiar to you?). There were days when he just sat and stared into space and I read or chatted (for what seemed like endless amounts of time) just to fill the air with sound. I learned never to take his mood swings personally. I learned to look past the day-to-day feelings and try to focus on the beauty of what we brought to each other's lives. My life today is truly rich because the Universe presented itself to me in a way that I was never expecting. I learned a million little things from being a caregiver. I learned to celebrate how blessed my life is because of giving to another.

For almost six years, I cared for this man and, during that time, I continued to learn and grow. About five years into the process, I began receiving phone calls from others who were facing similar situations with their parents. They were desperate for help and they had no time. I realized that there are thousands of professional caregivers who are able to work, but the missing link was someone to care for the family, someone to help them manage the unmanageable, and someone to coordinate life because they simply didn't have the time to do this. Because of this realization, I took the plunge and founded The Care Company. The company was created with the commitment to provide creative, straightforward, harmonious life solutions for seniors and their families—the very things I needed when I first started caring for Bob—and to help people manage senior crises with a little less stress. My personal experiences with Bob, and time spent since then with numerous other families, have shown me that the need is real for substantive support for caregivers navigating a senior crisis, and there is comfort in knowing that you are not alone in this journey.

PART I

The Basics

Caring for Your Loved One

Watching the physical and mental deterioration of an elderly loved one is painful. You feel helpless. You worry about the person's daily welfare. There are signs everywhere, but you aren't sure what to do. You're startled by what seems to be a sudden loss of functionality—both physical and mental. And when memory loss becomes apparent, you are saddened and frustrated by the seeming lack of interest your loved one takes in conversations or even day-to-day living. A host of new problems becomes present and, if you are like most people, you don't have the time to spend "fixing" your loved one's life and yet you know something must be done. You don't want to insult or hurt anyone's feelings. You haven't had "the conversation" yet; that was always easier to avoid. Your siblings don't want to get involved, or your family can't seem to agree on the next step. What do you do and where do you begin?

In many ways the elderly are a generation in crisis. No one ever believed that modern medicine would be able to keep people alive for such a long period of time. Most in this generation did not plan financially or emotionally, and this is where it gets difficult. Just because someone is alive, does not automatically mean that person has quality of life. Quality of life is key to the human condition.

When a family is spending all their time taking care of or looking out for the well being of the senior members, there is little or no time left to enjoy that person in a social capacity. Seniors have a great deal to offer, but it is often overshadowed by their personal frustrations and the fact that they do not want to be a burden on their family. They also have pride and don't want to be told what to do or how to do it.

As a society we often treat seniors or those with a handicap as though they have some kind of a disease. We don't reach out. We don't hug. We don't hold hands. I have no idea why this is, but I can tell you this—when someone is struggling with life challenges be they physical, emotional or mental; the one thing that they need more than almost anything else is the gift of touch. Sometimes all you need to do is just sit quietly and hold someone's hand. Touch a person's head or stroke an arm and suddenly the human connection exists and the world is just easier to deal with. When you become frightened or frustrated, try reaching out and holding your loved one's hand. You need not say a word; just let the human touch help both of you.

You will notice that much of the information contained in this book does not just apply to those caring for an elderly loved one. There is valuable information that can be utilized if you are a caregiver for anyone. The information in the self-care section of the book is especially pertinent for anyone living in this role. Many of the forms can also be used when keeping records. As a caregiver you are forever completing forms for someone or some institution. If you keep yearly copious notes and records, you will find that your work is not as tedious from year to year.

There are many things that can be done to make life safer and easier for your loved one and, at the same time, maintain their dignity, which in turn alleviates the pressure on the family. This care guide will help you understand, organize, and begin the thinking process about the next steps involved in caring for your loved one. Included in this manual is a section dedicated to self-care. It is absolutely essential to remember that a sick caregiver is no caregiver at all. Self-care is not selfish, nor should you think of it that way. This is a journey that you will travel with your loved one. You need to be at the forefront of that journey. If you learn how to indulge in self-care throughout the journey, you will reap all the soulful rewards that come to those who give to another human being.

Remember—it's a journey and you are the guide.

The Signs

Most people suspect something is amiss with an elderly loved one long before they do anything about it. When you first suspect that something is wrong, you need to pay attention. There will be signs, some of which are: a dirtier house, unusual clutter, clothes that are not getting laundered or cleaned regularly, bills that haven't been paid or attended to in proper fashion, broken or dilapidated appliances, a lack of attention to personal hygiene, or an overall unkempt appearance in all areas of life. The refrigerator may contain rotting food or perhaps no food at all. If there is a pet, perhaps it hasn't been attended to for a while. If your elderly loved one is still driving, there might be dents or scrapes on the sides of the car or on the bumpers.

As alarming as this may be for you, it is just one more symptom that change is occurring.

If there is help in the house, it is possible that the staff has not been properly caring for your loved one. Oftentimes things will go missing, or your loved one won't be receiving the attention that was once given prior to memory loss or physical ailments. If this is happening, it is imperative to rectify the situation immediately. You must have help in the house that you trust to take care of your loved one and who will take proper care of the home. This is not an easy task. We often do not properly vet the people who we bring into our homes (more on this later).

Check the house carefully and make notes on anything that you observe or find missing. Do not get frustrated, and do not point out to your loved one that you have observed these things. You will only end up frustrating your loved one, and there is nothing that he/she can do about it. It's happened, and you have to move forward and begin rectifying the situation. Engaging in this type of conversation only adds stress to the situation for everyone involved. Think about what you would accomplish by pointing out a messy house in disrepair—shame, defensiveness, sadness, frustration. Absolutely nothing positive. The reality is that most people don't want to live this way, but they don't know how to solve the situation. This becomes your charge.

What to Expect

Once you have recognized that your loved one is in need of assistance, do not be upset if your good intentions are met with resistance. Most older people do not like change and do not want to be reminded that they need help. Approach change gently. When we find ourselves in this situation, we want to "fix it" and fix it *now*! Granted, you have to move quickly, but you need to have a plan. You can't rush in and change everything. The first thing to do is make sure the house is safe. At the end of the manual is a scavenger hunt (you remember those) that will walk you through all you need to do to elder-proof the home. A safe house is a place where accidents are kept at a minimum. A safe house means less time in the hospital. The reality is that one in every three seniors over the age of sixty-five will fall. Elder-proofing the house is a must.

It's time to have "the conversation." You probably know your loved one better than anyone else but, in my experience, approaching the subject from a loving, kind, and concerned place is the best way to begin. I like to make an appointment. Most people take appointments seriously and this is a serious conversation. Take your time and let your loved one know that you want him/her to be safe. Explain the reasons why safety is a concern of yours. Be clear about the falling issue. Falling is often the biggest fear that our elders secretly worry about. "What happens if?" is often the question. Just because it hasn't been brought up, doesn't mean it's not a real concern.

The most difficult challenge for many is the role reversal. It's so hard to think of being the go-to person for a parent or loved one. Our parents are the ones who are supposed to care for us. We are never really prepared for this transformational time in our lives, and there is no way to plan for the feelings that naturally occur. I've seen all the different reactions. There is often anger, because of the new inconvenience. There can be anger because of years of unresolved emotional issues. There is frustration because of the challenges that the family has to face. There is sadness (mostly on the part of women, especially if they are presumed to be the obvious caregiver) at the loss of the connectedness of a parent. Very few people are able to deal with this from an objective, non-emotional place. Give yourself a break. This is a journey; trust that you will find your way.

I learned a little trick along the way, and I'm a big believer in sharing life's little tricks to help others. If you find yourself getting really frustrated and about to lose your temper (yelling at your elderly loved one is *not* an option and solves nothing), try this: Go to a place where you can be a *Distant Observer*. Put yourself in your loved one's place and imagine how you would feel. Imagine the loss of independence. Imagine the feeling of each day being a huge physical and mental challenge. Imagine how it feels to not remember. Imagine going to doctors constantly. Imagine the things that you and I take for granted as presenting enormous challenges. Now do you understand why the elderly are often so crabby?

So here's what you do. Take yourself out of the fray. Consciously think about rising above the situation and looking down. You're there and so is your loved one, but you're not engaged. Suspend judgment. Take a breath and let your intelligent mind take over. Remove the emotion. Stay calm and take one issue at a time. You will not cover all the subjects you want to, so be clear about one or two things you want to check off the list. By doing this simple exercise, you remove yourself from the conflict; you are able to be compassionate and you won't take personally anything that might be said in frustration. If your good intentions are welcomed, consider yourself lucky.

Often families have internal conflict. If you have siblings, you might be met with resistance from them. Not everyone will necessarily agree that your elderly parent or relative is in need of care. Sadly, many families do not want to spend any extra money or time on a parent. It's just the way it is and, chances are, no amount of cajoling, or pleading, or making someone feel guilty, is going to make a difference. However, someone in the family needs to be in charge of the situation.

Nothing is worse for an elderly person than to think that he/she is responsible for family fighting. Whatever the differences are, *do not* argue about these things in front of the elder. That will cause stress, depression, sadness, and even illness. *Decisions need to be made based on what is in the best interests of the elder and then the rest of the family.*

Do not make too many changes too quickly. If your loved one lives at home, you must respect that things have been done in a certain way "forever" and this is very important for his/her comfort level. Don't rearrange their home just because you think it would be easier for them. Even though we are living much longer and longer, the aging process is not easy, especially when the body breaks down and every day it becomes more difficult to remember things that seemed like second nature just a short time ago. *Have compassion.* If you are short on patience, leave the room, take a breath, and come back. You don't want your intentions misinterpreted, but you also don't want to be perceived in a threatening manner. *Any new change feels threatening.* Remember that change is hard, even when it is meant to help. Ease into this process. Take your time with this process to set the stage for how your move forward.

Day-to-Day Living

Change is difficult for most people, but especially the elderly. They rely on consistency and stability. Because so much about their physicality or cognitive abilities are changing, it is imperative that a routine be established in the house. (See Appendix on The Daily Plan.) Each day should begin at approximately the same time and other daily tasks should follow in the same order, i.e. breakfast at a certain time, nap time, exercise, snacks, lunch, television shows, and reading. Whatever fills the day should be scheduled and shared with the senior. This is especially true if the senior is having a difficult time remembering. *Surprises cause anxiety.*

Do not, under any circumstances, think that unannounced doctor visits or appointments or even social visitors will be met with an affable attitude. Flexibility is not part of the aging process. Be gentle and casual, and simply state what will be happening on a daily basis. If nothing is scheduled, then the senior will assume that it is a normal day at home. Generally speaking, this creates a sense of calm. Too many new situations cause anxiety. Do not think that you need to fill the day with activities. Sometimes peace and quiet combined with comfort are all that are needed.

A good idea is to record outings and the senior's reaction to them. If you find something that brings pleasure, by all means schedule it again, soon. Keep track of doctor appointments that bring the most angst. When you revisit the same doctor, you will be able to let the office know in advance so they will be able to create a calm and caring environment for their patient. It is your responsibility to create an environment that is as stress free as possible. This is easily done with advance preparation and taking the time to communicate.

The Power of Touch

No prescription medication can take away loneliness or the feeling of isolation. There may be no words that can make an elderly or ill person feel better, but non-verbal connections, such as a kind touch, can make an elderly person feel as though you care in a way that words, or even deeds, cannot. Often, the elderly do not want to talk and this can be frustrating to a caregiver who is spending days on end doing things for a loved one. Try not to take silence personally. When things around the elderly are moving at a rapid pace, it can be difficult for them to keep up; so they go quietly into their thoughts, which are usually in the past. You don't have to have conversation to make a connection. A hug, a hand or shoulder massage, an offer to comb or brush the person's hair, or holding someone's hand can make all the difference in the world. Human beings all need to experience human touch until the end of our lives. Old skin is just that—old skin. Unless someone has a skin infection or a contagious disease, there is no reason to avoid physical contact.

So often I went to visit Bob and he was completely non-communicative. He usually sat in his chair with his eyes closed. There were days when I had maneuvered traffic, left meetings early to visit him, cancelled personal appointments because he needed me, or ignored my own needs just to be with him and, when I arrived, I was met with closed eyes and no communication. On those days, I never even got a "hello" or "goodbye." The first few times this happened, I was full of anger, beyond frustration. *Why was I called? What was I supposed to do that the caregiver couldn't do?* One day I arrived at his house and he was silent, and the silence was deafening. I was about to start yelling (purely out of frustration), when he opened his eyes and said, "Will you hold my hand and watch this movie with me?" And in that moment, I got it—again.

Do you ever notice how when the elderly walk, they often take a companion's arm or hand? I used to think it was for balance, security, stability; but I now believe that it's also for the human touch—the connection. Not everyone is comfortable with hand-holding. If you are one of these people, try rubbing or patting someone's shoulder or touching a knee when you are seated next to your loved one. You need to do what is comfortable for you, but human touch is better than most of the medicine the elderly receive.

Nursing home residents often feel so isolated and alone. Doctors and nurses are in and out of the room all day long, but very few have the time, or take the time, to make the touch connection. Imagine, if you can, what touch means to you. What is it like for you when someone holds you or caresses your face or places a supportive hand on your back? Imagine what that feels like for you. Imagine not having it. On those days when you are exhausted, try just being quiet, holding your loved one's hand, and let the positive feeling flow between the two of you. We all need to be touched. Allow yourself to see past the dementia or the Alzheimer's or the wrinkled skin or the lost eyes, and try to see the soul that still appreciates a human connection. You won't regret it.

Taking the Keys Away

Driving is a privilege and not a right granted to us by the United States Constitution. I am asked about the subject of driving more often than anything else. We tend to make this subject way more difficult than it needs to be. Again, there are signs everywhere that your senior loved one should not be driving. This is a serious issue and you must pay attention to it. There are obvious and subtle signs. Check your loved one's car. Are there dents? Are there scrapes? What condition is the car in? How are the tires?

Are there scrapes on the fence, garage door or the mailbox? What does the interior look like? How is the car parked? If you notice anything unusual about the car, ask what happened? If your loved one looks at you like you're crazy, then the chances are good that he/she has no recollection of anything happening.

Take a drive with the senior and gauge for yourself. Does the senior seem disoriented, uncomfortable, nervous or fearful while on the road? Does the senior appear to be aware of all the traffic, including pedestrians? Does the senior know where he/she is going? Is your loved one moving with the traffic, staying inside the lane or even hitting the curb when turning the car? Is he/she having a hard time paying attention to traffic lights or road signs. Is the senior staying out of the bike lane? What happens when an unexpected situation occurs? Does the senior daydream or become easily distracted? What happens if other drivers begin honking? Does the senior become angry or frightened. What happens in a parking lot? Is the senior able to park within the lines? Are you comfortable or are you holding to the door for dear life? Would you let your children drive in the car with your loved one, or is that just too unthinkable?

If any of the above scenario rings true for you, then you need to step in and make a change. It's a difficult conversation to have, but the alternative is not anything you want to have to think about. You need to choose your words carefully and with sensitivity, but you must act and act quickly. Losing the ability to drive impacts a person's independence as well as the person's dignity. It's very important that you have done your research before you have the conversation. Before you make the push to take away the keys, find alternative methods of transportation—family, friends, local programs, senior transportation services, etc. Often we avoid having the talk because we fear that one more thing is going to fall in our lap. It doesn't have to be this way. You can make arrangements for transportation that doesn't involve you.

I was speaking to a gentleman just recently and he was telling me that his ninety-four-year-old mother was still driving and that it made his siblings and him very nervous, because she needs oxygen 24/7, but when she drives she doesn't use it. Now, to anyone hearing story, the answer is fairly obvious. If the woman isn't using her oxygen, what happens if she becomes light-headed or passes out? If she's not using her oxygen, then her brain is not operating at full capacity. However, the reason given for not taking the keys away was that the family was afraid to discuss this with her. She is apparently feisty and very independent. I pointed out to him that there was not just a possibility of an accident, but the odds were not in her favor. The last thing a family wants is a law suit—and there will be one if an accident occurs when a senior should not have been driving.

Driving laws are different from state to state and many states, due to the influx of drivers, do not require a written or vision test except for every five years. And no driving test is even required! Too many people, not enough time. Consequently, the responsibility falls on you.

Let's assume that it's time to take the keys away. You've had the conversation and your loved one becomes belligerent and won't budge. You've presented transportation alternatives, but still no movement. If the senior doesn't believe that there is a problem, then it's not going to matter if you speak about your worries, traffic violations resulting in tickets, possible accidents, lawsuits, or even injury. Sadly, this is where most people give up, throw their hands in the air and figure that there is nothing that can be done about this. You still have options and one of them will work.

If you are getting nowhere, you should seek the assistance of the primary care physician. For whatever reason, seniors listen to doctors. Explain your concerns and be very clear about them. Don't sugarcoat anything. You need the doctor's help. Ask the doctor to speak to your loved one. If this doesn't work, contact your loved one's insurance company and explain your concerns. Insurance companies do not want to pay for unnecessary accidents. The insurance company can request actual driving, written, and visual tests to determine if the senior is able to continue being covered on the current insurance policy. (It's hard to believe that this is not part of the insurance process, but you have to reach out and request it.) If all else fails, contact the DMV and speak to someone about your concerns. They will request a test for the senior and take the license away. This all seems callous and unfair, but the reality is that we live in a very litigious society and there are plenty of attorneys out there waiting for something to happen. Don't let this happen to your loved one. Once the license is gone and there are no further insurance payments, you can funnel the money saved into transportation for your loved one.

Personal Interests

A senior's life is comprised of a wealth of history, traditions, customs, beliefs, and special interests. If at all possible, it is vitally important to nurture and continue to make these activities a part of life. Imagine how difficult it would be for you if you could not visit with friends, worship as you want, or spend time in a social environment. It's possible that your loved one might not be able to play a round of golf any longer, but you can make it possible for him/her to visit friends at the golf course. If your mother likes to shop and go to lunch, get creative and make it happen as often as possible.

Religious beliefs and customs are part and parcel of life for many seniors. Whether it's church, synagogue, mosque, or another place of worship, find a way for your loved one to continue a spiritual practice. Even if it's a quiet meditation in a garden each day, schedule this into the daily or weekly plan.

If the senior has certain hobbies or passions, make a record of this (see appendix for form) so that anyone from the outside will know what those interests or hobbies are. Engaging the senior in personally enjoyable activities keeps the spirit alive and the brain active. For example: Bob had a huge world map on the wall of his office and he would take any new person into the room and show them all the places he had traveled with his wife of sixty-two years. His face lit up and, after he visited the map, he wanted to look at photo albums. He truly came alive during these times.

You have to figure out what is going to make a difference. It might be photos or books or movies or music; but if you can bring the past to life, the result is peace and comfort.

Holidays

Holidays are critical in a senior's life. Inclusion and socialization are very important. Holidays conjure up all kinds of memories and can send someone into a downward spiral or, worse, into a deep depression if not handled with sensitivity. Memories can be an especially sensitive issue. They have the ability to be wonderfully moving if the senior is encouraged to share memories and experiences. However, if the senior is made to feel like his/her memories don't matter, a feeling of isolation can take over. Try not to let this happen. The more you can involve your loved one in holiday celebrations, the better.

There is something quite lovely about children learning from seniors. They carry our history in their souls and, unless someone has severe dementia or Alzheimer's, children can learn volumes about their culture, heritage, family traditions, etc., from an elder member of your family. Encourage the sharing of remembrances from long ago. The stories will warm everyone's heart. If you know that the senior has special traditions, try to include them into your holiday celebration. If it's a special food, or song, or gift, anything, a small amount of energy can reap a huge reward. Holidays are about making those we love feel loved. Don't leave your senior relative out of the festivities.

Gift-giving

Have you ever agonized over what gift to give your mom or dad or elderly relative? If you're like most of us, then the answer is: Yes. I remember so clearly wondering what to buy, so I put it off because I didn't know—and Bob already had everything, not to mention that he didn't do much of anything, so what could I possibly give? I would give anything now if I had just one more birthday or holiday to shop for him. Sometimes lessons come to us when it's too late.

I am here to tell you—it doesn't matter. Here's a list of great gifts that will make a difference.

- Find a photo from your loved one's past. Have it cleaned up and framed. Memories create happy moments.
- Give a beautiful hankie to a grandmother.
- Give a tie to grandpa. A tie says, "We're going somewhere fancy one day soon."
- Give a music box with a favorite song.
- DVDs of movies from their past create hours of peaceful afternoons.
- CDs of favorite music—or better yet, create a CD especially for your loved one.
- Make a basket of favorite treats or, better yet, have your children bake something special.

When someone reaches true maturity, it's not the things—it's the thought. It's the moments with the family. It's the treasure of being with loved ones.

Keeping Informed

Remember that change causes anxiety in the elderly. This is also the case with both good and bad news. This is the time in a person's life when shelter from bad news just might be a good thing, especially if the situation is out of the senior's control and even more so if you will be handling the situation. (This is particularly true with monetary issues.) Suppose the senior has to pay a surprisingly large amount in taxes for one year. You will deal with the accountant or business manager; the senior has no way to increase personal wealth; nothing can be done to change the situation, and so the question becomes: do you discuss this setback with the senior? Or do you assume the emotional burden of this situation? I'm not saying that you should assume the financial responsibility, but you don't necessarily need to discuss it with your loved one.

The kindest and most compassionate thing for you to do is to handle the situation with professionalism and not discuss it with the senior. Nothing good can come of burdening your loved one with news that could potentially cause undue stress and emotional upset. The recommendation here is to discuss the situation with the professionals who have been handling the senior's finances and, if you still need a personal release, discuss the situation with someone who can offer you comfort. Taking care of a loved one's life is like running a business. You wouldn't share bad news with your employees; you would deal with it, and that is the case here.

Seniors oftentimes exhibit childlike behavior. This is one way of garnering attention, but also, as mental capacity diminishes, it may be the only way they know how to deal with day-to-day living. Think back to when you were a child. When bad things happened or bad news was presented to your parents, chances are good that they didn't share all the details with you. So it goes with seniors. A large part of your job is to protect them from situations that are out of their control.

Doing Uncomfortable Things

One of the most challenging parts of the caregiving process is dealing with the really uncomfortable things that you might have to do. One never even considers bathing a parent or helping with toileting, but that comes with the territory. The aging process is not kind.

As seniors age the sense of smell declines and thus, many seniors are not aware of body odor or how a lack of personal hygiene presents itself to others. Due to the fact that bathing becomes less of a pleasure and more of a physical challenge, many seniors simply stop bathing. Clothing does not get laundered or sent to the dry cleaners and they begin to emit a very unpleasant odor. Not only that, but incontinence happens. Accidents happen, and once again, you need to help your loved one deal with this additional sign of aging. No one wants to do this. Almost fifteen to thirty percent of the senior population experience lack of urinary or bowel control and it's a source of embarrassment and other disturbing emotional issues. Many seniors withdraw from friends and family because they feel so ashamed. Many never even discuss the problem with their doctor. Many end up in assisted living facilities because families don't know what to do.

If you notice that your loved one is experiencing incontinence of any kind, make an appointment to see the doctor. There are medical treatments or medications that can help.

If there is a bowel issue, perhaps changing the diet or pre-scription medications can help. Enlist the doctor for support in this endeavor. You do not have to go it alone. If you have enlisted the help of the doctor and nothing has improved then it's time to begin using diapers. (I can feel you cringing at the thought of this.)

Diapers should be use as infrequently as possible, because seniors become easily dependent on them. If you need to, remind the senior about using the toilet. You can purchase a device that sits on top of the toilet seat and raises it for easier access. You can also have a plumber come in and add elevation to the existing toilet. Place a grab bar by the toilet for safety. In the beginning, try having your loved one wear a diaper in public and see how that works. This is a dignity issue. You do not want your loved one experiencing embar-rassment if it can be avoided. Assuming you've been to the doctor and the senior is fully aware of the problem, then dis-cussing diaper-wearing will not be an issue. However, there are ways to do this; Do not use the word diaper. Diapers remind us of babies and helplessness. Rather use the word undergarment, pad, shield or even underwear. Go to a medical supply store and speak to a representative about the undergarment made which is the easiest to use. They change constantly and now there are "pull up" diapers, which are the simplest. Even though the senior is wearing one of these diapers, encourage the use of the bathroom rather than the diaper. This is critical in avoiding "diaper dependence."

If your loved one is more incapacitated and needs help changing the diaper, by all means, do this in the privacy of the bathroom. Avoid facing the senior and adopt a nonchalant, nonjudgmental attitude. (It has to be done and after a few times, it won't be so bad. We humans adjust to many difficult circumstances in our lives.) Try to act casual (even if you aren't) and just go to your higher place. Tell yourself that cleaning the senior's bottom is just another chore, and tell your loved one that it's no different than cooking a meal or taking care of other details. Acknowledge the senior's embarrassment in a kind and loving way. Maintain the dignity of the senior by not discussing his/her incontinence with others. (This is a great place to practice a little role reversal. How would you want this handled if it was you?) Try to keep your sense of humor, and remember that you've handled situations that were far more unpleasant and challenging than this.

Showering is another odd thing to consider, but everyone needs to bathe, especially seniors who are susceptible to skin conditions. Unfortunately, showering often becomes a chore, rather than a pleasant part of the day. There are things you can do to make showering a less stressful experience. Purchase a shower chair from a medical supply store. While you're there, get a good, solid shower mat, a hand-held shower hose and some grab bars. If the senior can sit down and bathe by using the hand-held nozzle, then showering becomes much easier. Grab bars make the in and out safe and easy. If you are still worried about the safety of your loved one, then have the senior shower when you come to visit. The senior can take a shower, while you wait in the bathroom or outside the door to help with the safety issues. On days when showering is not possible, give the senior a sponge bath. You wash as much of the body as possible and let the senior wash his/her own private parts. You need to just make sure that the private areas are being properly cleaned. Personal hygiene is extremely important.

Once the shower or bath is over, then you want to pat the skin dry and immediately apply a moisturizer on the body. (Use one without alcohol as it dries out the skin.) If you have a senior who has more serious skin issues, you should seek the advice of a dermatologist for the best lotions to use. I am a huge advocate for Cabot POL (pure ointmental lipids) Cream. It is distributed by Cooperlabs in Ventura, California. I have seen this cream work wonders on fragile, irritated skin.

The truth is that there are going to be many issues that arise regarding the personal care of your senior loved one. The way you handle this is going to make all the difference. If you find that you are simply incapable of performing these duties, then you might want to consider bringing in a companion or a caregiver for a few hours a week to do the bathing and showering. I have faith, however, that together, you and your senior loved one will work through this process and create solutions that work for both of you.

Handling Medical News

As months or years go by, the senior's medical condition will inevitably change. You must decide if you are going to share all medical news as it comes along. This decision should be based on many factors:

- Is the senior mentally capable of comprehending medical information?
- Is the senior capable of emotionally processing medical information, especially if it isn't good news?
- Is the senior's functionality going to change? And if so, how much?
- Is the senior's routine going to change?
- Will new doctors or medical procedures be involved in the care process?
- Is pain going to be associated with the change?
- Will there be new medical protocols?

Each of these questions must be addressed before your decision is made. If the change is going to be minor, sometimes it is best keep information to yourself. You should discuss the medical change with the doctor and determine *together* what is in the best interests of the senior. Sometimes it's best to assume the burden yourself in an effort to avoid worrying the senior. Seniors have a lot of down time and their minds tend to wander to the darkest places of fear and worry.

If you are dealing with a senior who is fully cognizant, but ignores doctors' orders (especially when it comes to taking medications), you will have to be firm. Begin with gentle coaxing. Chances are good that your efforts will be met with a smile, an acknowledgement of what you want done, and a thank you for caring. Once you are gone, the senior does whatever he/she wants to do.

This is when you need to play "hard ball." If the senior is simply being stubborn about the new medical protocol, you have to step in.

Determine what the senior's goals are. Ask. You may not like the answer, but in order to have an intelligent conversation, you must ask the question.

Let the senior know exactly what is going to happen, physically or emotionally, if the protocol isn't followed. (For example: "If you don't take your Lasix, your ankles will swell, your edema will worsen, and the fluid will back up in your body, causing your breathing to become labored.) You will have done your research prior to this conversation so that you can speak intelligently to the issue.

If you don't get your point across, or the senior's behavior becomes more stubborn, you might need to ask for the assistance of the doctor. An amazing thing happens when you mention the doctor. This is a generation that believes in the sanctity of the doctor. Their word is "gold."

There is only so much you can do. There is only so much responsibility you can bear and, if the senior does not change, then you should leave it alone, explore all your options, walk away, and broach the subject at another time.

Caring for one's self is a sign of mental well-being. If all signs are indicating that the senior is not caring for his/her home, personal hygiene, nutrition, and medical care, this might be a time to consider hiring a caregiver. (See Selecting a Caregiver following The Medical Team in this notebook.)

The Medical Team

Know the primary care physician. This is a critical component when caring for the elderly. More than likely, there will be a team of doctors looking out for your parent or your senior friend or relative. The primary care physician should be the "quarterback" of this team. It is imperative that you trust this physician's reputation, because the primary care physician will recommend all other doctors on the "team." Once all the proper legal paperwork is in place, make an appointment to meet with this doctor, either alone or with the senior you are caring for. Advise the doctor that you will be overseeing the care and treatment for the senior, and ask the doctor to bring you up to speed on the condition of the patient.

At this time, you should have completed all the medical information sheets contained in the Appendix of this manual. An organized caregiver receives a warmer response from the doctor.

Doctors have precious little time, but this meeting is necessary even though some resent it. Doctors, for the most part, don't like answering a lot of questions. They are accustomed to giving information, but usually in modest doses. *The success of this meeting is contingent on your attitude.* You must be clear, respectful, and show great concern for the senior in question. Ask for the doctor's medical diagnosis. Have specific questions written down. You will appear prepared for the meeting and this will help you attain the information that you need.

This meeting is going to happen only once. It is possible that you may be charged for this meeting. Neither Medicare nor supplemental insurance typically pays for consultations; however, this is between the doctor and you. That being said, it is too important to allow the cost to be a deterrent if you have a choice. Indicate that you intend to pay for the doctor's time and that your time is flexible. Be accommodating. Remember, your goal is to acquire much-needed information so that you can reinforce the doctor's orders and achieve the goal for the best possible care.

For example: If the senior in question has high cholesterol and a heart condition and is eating bacon, eggs, and toast with butter for breakfast, this is clearly counter-productive to aid in the reduction of cholesterol levels or prevention of future heart disease.

Bring a list of all the senior's medications and ask the doctor to explain what each medication is for and what side effects might be expected. You should also ask about how all the medications interface with each other. If the primary care physician does not have these answers, ask for the name of a pharmacologist to assist with this process.

Pharmacologists investigate how drugs and chemicals interact with biological systems. Their aim is to understand drugs and their actions so they can be used effectively and safely. Some pharmacologists also carry out research to aid drug discovery and development. A good pharmacologist is an excellent resource. Don't be surprised if Medicare does not pay for a pharmacologist. But such a consult is well worth the investment. If you cannot locate a pharmacologist, find a good 24-hour pharmacy that you can consult if you have questions regarding medications. Pharmacists are usually very happy to work with a family, especially one that is doing their due diligence.

Do not be alarmed if the primary care physician is unaware of all the medications that the senior is taking. Many doctors do not confer with one another until someone (you) enters the scene and requests that the primary care physician oversee the team of doctors, i.e. cardiovascular, neurological, urologist, ophthalmologist, etc.

If you do not receive a positive response from this meeting, you may want to consider changing doctors. Just because the senior has been seeing the same doctor for a long time does not mean that the best care has been provided. Take your time to research your options. It is likely that you will be dealing with the doctors regularly, especially as the senior becomes less independent; so a good relationship between you and the doctor(s) is of the utmost importance. A good medical team is vital.

The hospital that the senior's doctors are affiliated with is an important consideration. You must be comfortable with the hospital, the staff, its reputation, its emergency room, and its location. *Do the research.* Appropriate hospital care becomes increasingly more important as someone ages or as a condition worsens.

If you decide to make any medical changes, be sure to discuss this with the senior. Explain the reasons you feel a change is necessary. *Again, do the research.* Check with friends about their doctors or the doctors who care for their parents.

This should not be a quick process. Interview doctors to make sure that you and the doctor have a good rapport, and that the doctor understands your family's situation.

Do not assume that your opinion is going to be valued by your elderly loved one. You must have valid reasons for your decision. Once you find a replacement primary care physician, schedule a meeting for an exam with the senior. At this time, let the senior know that you are going to another doctor to get a second opinion. It will be an easier transition for everyone, because, if you recall, change causes anxiety. Even if the change is in the senior's best interest, there will still be angst. The comfort factor always wins.

Selecting a Caregiver— Buyer Beware!

Making the determination that an elder relative or friend is in need of an outside caregiver or nurse can be an anxiety-provoking task. There are hundreds of companies claiming to have the most capable, patient, kind, and trustworthy caregivers. There are vast pricing differences and with those differences comes an equally vast difference in quality of service. You must approach this task as you would any business transaction. The safety of your loved one and the security of the home depend on it. Research. Interview. Interview some more. Request recommendations and ask to see a current license. It seems easy, right? Well, it's not. Too many people panic and hire the first or second person who comes along. They lose their perspective and, consequently, make quick and often rash decisions.

Let me tell you that hiring professional help, even if it's for a few hours a week, is a great way to offset some of the stress that accompanies family caregiving. However, you must be cautious. Have you ever noticed how amazing it is that when people make a decision to adopt a dog or cat from a rescue organization, they're required to answer endless questions about themselves and their family? And the answer is sometimes a resounding, "I'm sorry, but you don't meet the criteria for adoption." Kudos to the animal rescue for their thoroughness, but the irony here is that we're often not nearly as thorough in screening the people who will care for our loved ones.

Finding a caregiver requires that you do some research and work. If you are willing to do this, the payoff is going to be huge for your family and your parents. There are wonderfully compassionate caregivers in need of work, but alternatively, there are some real predators out there and you do not want to bring them into your loved one's home or you'll be heading into a real disaster. Let me guide you through the process of selecting a caregiver.

Do Your Homework

Hundreds of agencies represent caregivers. The best way to select one is via a referral. Do an extensive interview on the phone and, if possible, meet with the owner of the company in advance. Be sure to ask about the owner's experience and qualifications with caregiving. *This is really important.* It's important that you let the owner of the caregiving company know that you are in control of this process. Due to the huge demand for caregivers in this country, many people are jumping onto the bandwagon without ANY previous experience. Find a company that is owned and operated by someone who has been in the caregiving business with personal case experience.

Implement a Thorough Screening Process

Once you have selected a company, ask to interview several caregivers and make sure that you are doing a background check on all of them. Ask for fingerprints, a resume and references. Contact their references. No excuses about this. Personality plays a major role when selecting a caregiver for your loved one. Even if you are in a huge hurry to find someone, you really need to slow down and take your time to find the right person. By doing this, you will avoid hours of work for yourself. If a candidate finds this process offensive, move on. We're talking about your loved one's safety and well-being and you must be a soldier about this. Remember, your goal is to find a caregiver whom you trust with your family or loved ones. Trust takes time. Be cautious and careful and remember that caregivers often have very limited training and are not required by law to have a license. A caregiving course can be completed in a weekend. (We require more certification from fitness trainers!) Ask about experience in addition to references.

Outline Specific Responsibilities and Expectations

What should caregivers be expected to do? It is unreasonable to think that they will be able to provide any kind of care beyond simple, low-maintenance needs such as basic hygiene, meal preparation, and cleaning. Moreover, they are generally not professionally trained in medical treatment procedures and emergency circumstances other than CPR. Unfortunately, due to a lack of understanding by the family about limitations, many caregivers are expected to administer medical modalities such as providing wound care, gauging blood pressure medications, assessing and interpreting vital signs, etc. *In no way, are they trained to do this!* It frightens me when caregivers make medical decisions for patients without the fundamental knowledge of anatomy and physiology at the very least. Lack of knowledge often leads to a variety of physical side effects the patient unwillingly endures.

Be aware that caregivers are not regulated by the state. When they are engaging in activities that are way out of their scope of practice (basic custodial care), problems definitely ensue. There are real positives in having a support system for the elderly/patients so that they are not alone and are supported in basic needs, and you can have a break from the day-to-day responsibilities.

Caregivers are not even supposed to administer medications. Here's an example of what can happen. I was brought in to consult with a family after the following incident occurred: The family had hired a caregiver for their elderly mother and made the mistake of leaving things in the caregiver's hands. The mother was taking blood pressure medications. The caregiver took the patient's blood pressure and it was low. In response, the caregiver withheld the blood pressure medication, thinking this action would help lower the patient's blood pressure even further. Unfortunately the patient suffered a stroke because her pulse rose rapidly. The cardiac medication prescribed was for the pulse purpose, not just for the blood pressure. This was a nightmare, and an unnecessary incident resulted in the patient requiring hospitalization and a higher level of care upon her return home due to her stroke. She never fully recovered.

It's not fair to expect caregivers to ascertain the difference in pharmacology. These types of mistakes are made everyday, especially with the rise of polypharmacy, which simply means that multiple doctors are prescribing numerous medications and no one is monitoring them. As discussed before, this happens on a regular basis with the geriatric population. If you wish to have the caregiver administer medications, it's wise to put this in writing, sign it, ask the caregiver to sign it, and keep it in the caregiver's file. It is really a protection for the caregiver. Be specific about your intentions.

Assuming your goal is to ensure that your elderly loved one is properly cared for while you are provided with some relief, you must be diligent about selecting the caregiver who is best suited for your loved one's needs and personality, and who is going to interface the most effectively with you. You also must keep your perspective about the requirements of the position and not ask a caregiver to do more than they are trained and able to do. Take your time, do your research, follow this advice, and I assure you the rewards will be worth the investment.

For more information see the Caregiver Task List in the Forms Section of this manual.

Taking Care of Business Matters: Getting Life in Order

What to Do First?

Part of the process of providing caregiving for another is the understanding that you are basically running a small business. When the time comes for you to step in and handle the affairs of your loved one, you want to remove as much of the emotion as possible. Do what is necessary. There is plenty of time for emotion later.

Gather together the bills and important papers. Find the checkbook. Write out checks. Have your loved one sign them and get them in the mail immediately. It is a good idea to contact all creditors and explain the current situation. Let them know of any future changes that will be taking place. Assure the creditors that, going forward, they will be paid in a timely fashion. These phone calls work in restoring good faith and should definitely be made.

If things have deteriorated to the point where major bills are going unpaid, you might want to consider having someone in the family become the Power of Attorney for Limited Assets. If you have an attorney, it is a good idea to make contact and seek professional advice. This is a touchy subject and needs to be broached cautiously. Be aware that unless you have *written* Power of Attorney or are named as an Authorized Account Manager, credit card companies, doctors, nurses, government officials, mortgage account specialists, etc., are not legally able to talk to you; and no amount of prodding, pleading, or screaming will get them to speak to you. The Power of Attorney or Account Manager appointment is delicate and requires some serious thought on the part of the family and your loved one. If possible, do not omit your loved one from these discussions. Inclusion is critical for success in this situation. (This is assuming that the person for whom care is necessary has the cognitive ability to understand what you are talking about.) You must explain that the person who becomes their Power of Attorney is going to make life less complicated and smoother, but that your loved one will still be included in all business decisions.

Choose this person very carefully. Having a Power of Attorney requires time, patience commitment and trust. Assuming you have an attorney, a discussion about this is beneficial. You really need to keep emotions out of this decision. Ultimately the person who is selected should be willing to perform the duties that accompany this responsibility. As the senior's health and faculties change, the responsibility becomes more profound. Enter into this carefully.

Remember that a Power of Attorney for Finances is different from a Durable Power of Attorney for Health. It might very well be that more than one person is involved in this process.

Protecting Your Loved One

No time should be wasted in putting the necessary protections in place. Situations have occurred where a household employee convinces the senior or friend that life would be easier if the employee was able to pay bills or have the authority to charge on credit cards. If your elderly relative gives the bank or credit card companies the authority to do this, even if under duress, and someone from the family is not listed as a contact in case of changes to accounts, entire bank accounts can and have been wiped out.

Protect your loved one and your family. It is difficult to imagine the atrocities that take place and the abuse that is often inflicted on unsuspecting, trusting seniors who are in need of care. You need only to read the paper or listen to the nightly news to become enlightened. Do not think that this is something that only happens once in awhile. It is a regular occurrence in our country and, as sad and horrifying as it seems, many of these people never get caught.

Be careful. Be present. If you have outside help in the house, you need to show up regularly and ask to see bank records, check books, and household receipts. It's a good idea to have a box in the kitchen where all receipts must be placed. Do not give outside help access to a credit card, even if you think it's a good idea and will cut back on your responsibilities. Temptation is a bad thing. If you think anything suspicious is going on, *make changes immediately.* Oftentimes, your loved one is aware that something isn't right, but is too afraid of being left alone or of upsetting the family to say anything. Even though change is difficult, in some cases it might be welcome. Follow your instincts.

A Quick Legal Lesson

Power of Attorney

A Power of Attorney is a legal document in which the elder family member gives another person legal authority to act on his/her behalf. The Power of Attorney might cover simple tasks such as writing or endorsing checks or more complicated matters like selling real estate or making legal decisions. The Power of Attorney can be specific to just one task, or a person can give the agent the power to do everything that he/she once did. Your attorney will be able to help the family understand how to tailor the Power of Attorney to fit the elder's wishes and needs.

Choosing the Agent

A person can give Power of Attorney to anyone. The agent does not have to be an attorney. Choose someone who is a trusted family member. Choose someone who can be gentle and patient with the senior. Be sure to have your lawyer draw up the necessary documents. (You can complete these documents yourself, but make sure that someone qualified looks them over.) Reassure the elder that the person who has Power of Attorney will not be taking over, but rather will provide a second set of eyes and a concerned and trusted opinion. The Power of Attorney may be revoked at any time.

Types of Powers of Attorney

There are four types of Powers of Attorney. The type of Power of Attorney selected will depend on the need and how much authority the elder family member wants the selected agent to have; when the agent should begin acting on the elder's behalf; and when, if ever, the Power of Attorney comes to an end.

Limited Power of Attorney—Through a Limited Power of Attorney, a person is authorized to do specific things for a limited amount of time. (For example, if a surgery is involved and the elder is incapacitated, a Limited Power of Attorney is the perfect solution and might provide peace of mind.) In general, the Limited Power of Attorney ends at a specified time.

General Power of Attorney—A General Power of Attorney gives another person the authority to do whatever the elder is not able to do. This is powerful and must be given very careful thought.

Durable Power of Attorney for Health—A Durable Power of Attorney for Health authorizes the chosen agent to continue to act for you after you become incapacitated, but ends upon the elder's death. It becomes effective as soon as it is signed. You must have a conversation with the senior and be very clear about the specific end of life care and decisions. This is such an important document and ensures that the senior receives the type of treatment that he/she desires. This document gives people their dignity.

Springing Power of Attorney—This document can be written so that it goes into effect only if the elder becomes incapacitated. With this Power of Attorney, you must be very careful to define exactly what the "springing" event will be.

Financial and Medical Powers of Attorney

It is a good idea to have separate Powers of Attorney for finances and healthcare. Within each legal document, the elder specifies the specific terms the chosen agent must follow in carrying out the elder's wishes. A durable Financial Power of Attorney allows the agent to carry out financial tasks for the elder when he/she cannot do so. This might include paying bills, managing property, or handling any and all money matters. A durable Medical Power of Attorney lets the chosen agent make medical decisions for the elder when he/she can't make these decisions any longer. Select this person very carefully.

What is An Advanced Health Care Directive?

Adults have the fundamental right to control decisions relating to their healthcare care. You have the right to make medical and other healthcare decisions so long as it is possible for you to give informed consent for those decisions. No treatment may be given to you over your objection at the time of treatment, including nutrition and hydration. You may decide whether you want life-sustaining procedures withheld or withdrawn in instances of a terminal condition. When a person is no longer able to make those decisions, and an Advanced Health Care Directive is not in place, no decision is made and quality of life is no longer an option. By law, doctors must keep a patient alive regardless of this person's preferences or desires.

As difficult as it is to think about the care and treatment you want in the event you should become incapable of making medical decisions on your own, an Advanced Health Care Directive will give you a voice even if you are rendered incapacitated. An AHCD allows individuals to appoint an agent who has Power of Attorney to make care and treatment decisions on their behalf, and give instructions about their healthcare wishes.

Once decisions have been made and the appropriate forms are completed, you will need to have them notarized. Copies of the completed forms should be given to each person named as agent, or proxy, and to an individual's primary care physician. Keep the original in a safe place.

*Note: The forms for the various Powers of Attorney are not included in this book as they vary from state to state. Be sure you acquire the proper forms for your particular state.

Securing Personal Information

Important Papers and Documents

Every household has important papers and documents. It may be necessary to go through file cabinets, a safe (if there is one), desk drawers, etc., and locate any important documents that should be removed from the home and brought to a safe location. Anything that includes the senior's identity, such as documents with social security numbers, driver's license, passport, access codes, deed to the house or any other property, and mortgage information, etc., should be gathered together and locked in a safe or, better yet, removed from the home. Identity theft is the fastest-growing crime in the United States. It happens when someone accesses essential elements of a person's identifying information in order to commit theft. This information includes name, address, Social Security number, date of birth, and mother's maiden name. Many identity thieves use this personal information to open credit card accounts, obtain loans, and even mortgages in the victim's name.

Identity thieves may use a variety of methods to gain access to someone's personal information, such as:

- Stealing records from their employer (Imagine the easy access household help has to your family member's identity.)

- Bribing an employee who has access to the records
- Conning the information out of employees
- Stealing wallets or purses
- Stealing mail, including bank and credit card statements, pre-approved credit offers, new checks or tax information
- Completing a "change of address form" to divert mail to another location; and/or
- Obtaining information directly from the unsuspecting individual just in simple day-to-day conversation

The possibilities are endless and reprehensible; however, this happens every day and seniors are more susceptible to this crime than the average citizen. Be diligent and protect your loved one.

Important Information and Contacts

If you are the victim of identity theft, do not assume that it's going to be resolved easily. The following is a list of numbers of companies who need to be contacted.

Credit Cards—Call the number on the back of the credit card, and report it immediately.

Stolen Checks or Fraudulent Bank Accounts—If your checks are stolen or you believe your bank account has been compromised, call the following companies after you have contacted your bank:

Certegy, Inc.
1-800-437-5120

TeleCheck
1-800-710-9898

SCAN
1-800-262-7771

Federal Trade Commission (FTC)
Identity Theft Clearing House
600 Pennsylvania Avenue NW
Washington, DC 20580
www.consumer.gov/idtheft
1-877-IDTHEFT

Social Security Administration's Fraud Hotline
P.O. Box 17768
Baltimore, MD
www.ssa.gov/org
1-800-269-0271

U.S. Postal Inspector
www.usps.gov/websites/depart/inspect
See your local telephone directory

Credit Bureaus

Equifax
To report fraud, call 1-800-525-6285, and write:
P.O. Box 740241
Atlanta, GA 30374-0241
www.econsumer.equifax.com
For a credit report call 1-800-685-1111

Experian
To report fraud, call 1-888-397-3742, and write:
P.O. Box 9532
Allen, TX, 75013
www.experian.com/consumer
For a credit report call 1-888-397-3742

TransUnion
To report fraud, call 1-800-680-7289, and write:
Fraud Victim Assistance Division
P.O. Box 6790
Fullerton, CA 92834-6790
www.transunion.com
For a credit report call 1-800-916-8800

End of Life Decisions

Americans plan for nearly every phase of life. We plan the birth of our children. We register them for preschool when they are just a few months old. We plan where we will live based on schools. We plan and save for college, and on and on—you get the picture, because chances are you're a planner. We plan our careers. Sometimes, we plan whom we will marry. We plan and plan and plan, but few of us plan for the end of our lives.

When I was caring for Bob and his wife, it became increasingly apparent that they had made no plans for end of life. Death was not something they ever thought about or even considered. She passed three years before he did and I was met with decisions that I never should have had to make. His despair over losing the love of his life made it all the more difficult. Initially I resented the position that had been placed in my hands. It didn't matter how capable I was; I didn't feel like I should be making these decisions. I had to guess about what she would have wanted, as in their sixty-plus years together they had never had the conversation. In the end, her funeral and the reception following were both beautiful; but I vowed I wasn't walking that road again.

I learned that I can vow all I want, but having the conversation with "him" was far more challenging. He wanted *nothing* to do with the subject. I loved his "I'm-going-to-live-forever attitude." Once he was diagnosed with a terminal illness, the conversation became necessary.

Each person is unique in the way this discussion is received. For some, it's all business and very factual. For others, it's too emotional to discuss and you need to find your way through the weeds. Be gentle and don't intrude. If the person is dramatic, play to that. "This is the final moment and all eyes are on you. How do you want the world to see you?" Know your senior. I was caring for a proud World War II veteran and I approached him with military-like questions. I asked him what he didn't want so we could arrive at what he wanted. He was *very clear* about what he did *not* want. I knew that he was unaware that he was entitled to a military burial and, when I asked him about this, he said nothing, but his eyes told the story. A military burial is a most moving experience and it is given to our veterans, provided that you have their discharge papers.

For many seniors, religion and faith have played a key role throughout their lives. Whether you believe or not, this is the one time when you need to honor their religious beliefs. And then there are seniors who did not practice any particular religion, nor did they believe in God. For this person, you can still have a spiritual ceremony, but not one that is rooted in religion.

Whatever it is that someone wants, you must try to honor it, even if it's not your choice. This is not your life we're talking about here. Be respectful by listening and acting. If possible, find a way to make it happen. Most seniors want to be celebrated when they leave this earth. Most want friends and family to know of all the richness of their lives. They have earned their place. Most are being freed from illness, dementia, Alzheimer's, or chronic conditions, and there is joy for them in the release. As difficult as this is for us to come to terms with, they really are at peace.

If the person or persons who will be delivering the eulogy has not already been selected, think about who will give the most rousing and loving send-off. If there are grandchildren, it's lovely to have them say something—something short, yet heartfelt.

This is your chance to give the final gift. Be resolute in making it happen.

See the Forms Section of this book for more information on organizing this emotional time in the family's life.

PART II

Personal Care:
Yes, You Matter!

Caring for Yourself

If you don't take care of yourself—who will? I learned about self-care the hard way. Because I was literally thrown into the caregiver role, and because I'm somewhat of a Type-A personality, I tackled this role with a vengeance. I was going to be the savior. I was going to "fix" everything that was wrong. I was riding in on the white horse to save the day! I don't know why caregivers think they can fix everything that is wrong, because you can't! It's illogical to think like this, and yet, I've never met a caregiver who doesn't share a common understanding of the "fix-it notion." I'm convinced it's part of the process, and you will come to understand the truth in this statement in your own time.

When you consider that the majority of seniors are being kept alive with numerous medications, it stands to reason that you will not be able to change the physical or mental decline that is happening to your loved one. But it's natural to try, and, I think, it's a beautiful component of the human condition that we want to help make someone well to the point when logic doesn't really enter the dialogue. Maybe we believe that if we can just fix it, we can somehow have our lives back. Maybe we believe because we want our loved one back the way he/she once was. However, the reality is that you probably can't fix anything. You can only act as an advocate and a companion. And do not disregard the value of being the person who provides this comfort.

Family caregivers fall into a couple of categories. Many are angry, angry at seeing the changes that are happening to their loved ones, angry at the perceived imposition on their lives, and angry at the world because reality is not always pleasant. Then there are those who are deeply saddened and become paralyzed by their sadness. They can't bear to see the changes taking place and because they feel so unprepared and inept at their new role, sadness takes over. And finally, there is a whole group of family caregivers who are living in denial. Denial is the most challenging for the medical community, because communication is next to impossible. This is the group that stays away. This is the group who find silly, insignificant things to focus on, i.e. a missing pair of bedroom slippers. All of these reactions are normal and part of the process. Most people have to work through the journey in their own way and time. Men often have a more difficult time with this process than women. It's just nature and the inherent differences between the sexes. Men approach life in a much more matter-of-fact way and thus, have a harder time with the eldercare process. Women, on the other hand, jump in, take over, and, because they are managing their personal lives, families, and often a career, tend to get consumed by the process. Finding balance is essential.

My story was typical. I spent hours on end at the hospital. I practically lived there and, when Bob came home, I was at his house round the clock in spite of the fact that he had full-time registered nurses caring for him. Somehow when I wasn't there, I felt guilty. When I was there, I felt guilty that I was ignoring my family and my responsibilities. Prior to leaving my career, I was unable to work, because I couldn't concentrate. I didn't sleep. I stopped exercising. I wasn't eating properly and, if the truth be told, I looked like hell. I snapped at everyone except him. I was his angel. He needed me, I thought, more than my husband, my own parents, and my daughter. This is never the case. What became painfully clear is that the more you give—the more you're expected to give, and it's like a merry-go-round that never stops to let you off. The day comes when you feel like you're on a runaway train, and that's when you're in trouble.

One day we were at a routine visit with one of his doctors and at the end of the visit the doctor asked to speak to me alone. I stayed back and Bob left the room with his nurse. The doctor looked at me and said, "You cannot fix what's wrong. You need to accept that and you need to live your life and take care of yourself. A sick caregiver is no caregiver at all." He went on to say that I was doing no one, including Bob any favors by killing myself. There would be many years of caring for him and he would need for me to be there through the entire journey. *Bingo! I finally got it.* I drove him home and left his house for four days! (This was a huge accomplishment for me.) And I took care of myself.

What did that look like? I began by crying for hours. I couldn't stop no matter how hard I tried. I felt like a baby. I cried for him. I cried for myself. I cried for my family. I cried for my lost career. I cried and cried and cried. I let myself feel the pain of caregiving. I had spent months stuffing my feelings and they came flooding out. Then I crashed and slept for hours in the middle of the day; something I hadn't done in years. When I finally woke up, I felt like a truck had hit me! I had been ignoring myself for so long that I became immune to the screams that were coming from my body and soul. I had stuffed my feelings for equally as long and I was totally tapped out. Two days turned into four, because I fell apart. After the first two days of rest and tears and sleep, I set out on a new path. Yes, I was a caregiver, but that role would not define me. I was no longer going to be consumed by the process. There would still be days and times of struggle, but I would save for those days, and I was going to be in control of this process. If any of this feels true for you, then I encourage you to check in with yourself. Get help if you need it and, whatever you do, don't shut the world out of your life.

The Process

For each of us, the process of self- discovery and honoring our needs is different. If the truth be told, I had never really done this before. I was a giver. I wanted everyone to like me (they didn't, but I wanted them to). I was like a baby learning to walk. The thought that I had needs and that I could ask for what I needed was a completely new concept for me. I was very adept at deluding myself and I was even better at making it look like I had it all together. The thing about "process" is that, once you begin, you really can't stop. The success of this is completely dependent upon how open or closed you are. I was open, because I had to be and I felt like the caregiving journey was handed to me from a Universal Power far greater than myself. My life had been turned upside down one too many times, and I had never done the work. This time I was hit over the head with a two-by-four! It was time to listen.

We are taught a lot of things in this life, but how many of us learn about boundary setting? It's not a course one takes in school. Most of our parents don't teach us this; because the truth is that most people don't understand about boundaries. Sure, we have rules that we follow. At work, we have an understanding about boundaries, but are they the company's or ours? For me, I had to learn about boundaries and I had to learn it in a way so that I would be heard without offending the world. I was great at smiling through pain and "sucking it up" as my dad would say, but when I was pushed to the end of my limits I was a holy terror! I shook my fist at the world like an agitated little child and no one listened. In fact, they turned away. It became a vicious cycle for me.

I approached this process like a business. The business had to have a plan and a usable one, so that I could follow it. It had to be adaptable to a life that often didn't include a plan. And it had to contain certain components: *Health, Wellness, Time Management, Personal Time, Social Time, Exercise,* and *Spirituality.* Those were my "musts," the things I could no longer live without. What does your list look like? Take a few minutes here and just get quiet and listen to the quiet of your soul. It will speak to you. Perhaps you've turned it off for so long that you don't know how to listen. If this is the case, stay quiet. Your soul will speak and usually in volumes.

Keep paper or a journal with as you as you do this exercise and write down whatever comes to mind. Allow your mind to run free. Write your thoughts, your personal needs, and even go out on a limb and write your personal desires.

I knew I wouldn't be able to succeed if I didn't have some boundaries in place. But I had no idea how to set them. Another exercise in patience and personal kindness was about to ensue. I began writing. This is my way of personal expression. How would I accomplish this? Somehow the answer coupled with clarity made its way to the page. The following is what I learned and I share with you. If you follow this formula, your life will be infinitely better. I encourage you to pass this on to your children. Our society will be far healthier if we learn a little boundary-setting.

Setting Boundaries to Save Your Sanity

Before we set boundaries, we *know* something needs to change, but change is not easy for us humans. We know why we need to lose weight, or why our bodies need exercise, or why we need to quit smoking. We also know when we feel like our lives are spinning out of control or when we feel helpless; but the question always becomes, "How do we make the change?" You know what it took for me. *What will it take for you?* In order to make a change, one that becomes the fiber of your existence, there has to be a meaning attached to it. For example, if you went to the doctor and were told that you had diabetes, you would know exactly what changes you needed to make to manage your illness. Your life change would become crystal clear and, more than likely, you would do it. So what is it about making personal life changes that is less clear? Perhaps it's because our *shoulds* seldom become our *musts*. When you make this transforming jump in your thinking, you gain new perspective. It's hard to argue with the musts in our lives.

As I've said before, it seems that for many of us, setting boundaries is the real challenge. Setting boundaries is the first step in self-care. We worry that if we nurture ourselves, we'll be perceived as selfish. We fear that we won't be liked. We don't think our opinions will matter. We even wonder if our children will stop loving us! Setting boundaries is HUGE for most people and sadly we don't even recognize that it is a large part of many of the frustrations that plague our lives.

People treat you as you allow them to and you can subliminally teach others (including your family members) to treat you based on the strength or weakness of your boundaries. Setting boundaries can have an enormous impact on the quality of your life. It is the first step in helping you create the kind of life you really want for yourself.

So how do you accomplish this? Ask yourself these questions.

- Do I agree to do things for others that I really don't want to do?
- Do I feel guilty when I put my needs first?
- Do I feel like I'm an easy target and that people are often taking advantage of me?
- Do I have resentment when I say "yes," but really mean "no?"
- Do I feel unappreciated, even though I feel like I'm always doing things for others?

These are some of the questions you should ask yourself as you begin the process of setting boundaries. If you answered yes to even a couple of them, then it's time to make a change.

Setting your personal boundaries is the first in many steps in helping you take back your life. It's the beginning of the process in defining yourself. Understand that when you don't have boundaries set, other people, including your loved ones, will easily step over the line without even realizing where the line is. This is not about getting others to change; rather, this is about the process of creating your best life. Perhaps you are nodding your head in agreement with all of this, but are wondering where to begin. Here's what I did that worked.

- Write down all of your pet peeves. Once you've completed this task, read through them, and ask yourself if any of the things that really bother you could be handled if you had set boundaries.

- Spend some time in your own self-awareness. Where do you need more space, self-respect, personal time, and energy? What makes you angry, resentful, frustrated, or powerless? Once your triggers are identified, you will see that a boundary has probably been crossed.

- Give yourself permission to begin honoring yourself and others in new ways. This is *not* about you changing others; it's about changing yourself. How would you like to improve your life? Would you like time to exercise? Would you like time to just be quiet for thirty minutes a day? Would you like to select the restaurant or movie with your friends, or would you like co-workers to respect your position at work as much as they do their own? Whatever your needs are, you must first define them and make a commitment to honor them. If you don't honor your new boundaries, then you can't expect anyone else to, either. Once you actually begin practicing this, others will, too, and you will become a much more attractive person to be with as your past anger and resentment will begin to dissipate.

- Set the example. If you want people to respect your boundaries, then you must respect theirs.
- Schedule time for yourself. If you want to exercise, schedule it into your calendar and stick to it. You must also learn to respect the boundaries that you set for yourself. If someone asks for your input, by all means, give it. It's easy to say, "I don't care," but you know that you really do. Don't fall back into your old ways.

Remember that your personal boundaries are valid and you don't need to defend, debate, or justify them to anyone. If a boundary is crossed, be courteous and graceful in your communication. Yelling about your boundaries is only going to create resentment. This is your path to your own serenity and joy. This is a new skill and you will have to practice it. Once a plan is created, you need to review it daily. You should understand that in the beginning, it's not going to be easy, but with time, you will make the necessary changes and you will begin to feel relief. If you falter, you will know it. The same feeling of helplessness and anger will reappear. Be aware of your internal feelings, give yourself a break and simply move forward. This is a process.

We have but one life to live. There are no do-overs. We don't get days back, but we always have the opportunity to change what isn't working for us. Caregiving is one of life's tasks that affords us numerous opportunities to become better, more vibrant human beings. It's all in how we handle the journey.

Caring for the Caregiver

It's a well-known fact that millions of Americans are suffering what is now termed as "caregiver burnout." Let's just go over the numbers once again. In the United States, 36,500,000 people are age sixty-five or older accounting for twelve percent of the population. Of those 36,500,000, almost five million are eighty-five and over. By the year 2050, it is expected that almost 87,000,000 people will be over sixty-five and comprise twenty-one percent of the population. This constitutes a 147 percent increase in the population of this age group. Most seniors with long-term care needs (65 percent) rely exclusively on family and friends to provide assistance. It's estimated that 59-75 percent of those caregivers are women, most of whom are married and work outside the home. Although men provide assistance, female caregivers spend as much as fifty percent more time providing care than male caregivers. Yes, the figures are astounding, and caregiving is here to stay. So we have to learn how to manage it.

We've previously discussed the caregiver "Fix-It Role" and, as a female caregiver, it is natural for you to be tempted to try and do *everything* for your loved one. Depending on the condition of your loved one's health, you may find yourself having to do many things they previously did for themselves, such as personal grooming (see chapter in Part One), driving to appointments, or day-to-day household duties. Responsibilities such as these have the potential to cause undue stress. Even if the person is greatly dependent upon you for their care, you will find that you are better able to maintain your own mental and physical health, and the dignity of the person for whom you are caring, if your roles and responsibilities are clearly defined. This is not the time to be shy about your needs. (Here come your boundaries.) It is the key to your survival, and you must clarify your role through open communication. Unless your loved one is mentally incapacitated, you must talk about their wants and needs, and be sure to make yours clear as well. Discuss today's necessities, but plan for the future. In time, you may find yourself with increased responsibilities such as, medical, home maintenance, legal, and financial matters. Make certain that you not only understand what your fiduciary boundaries are, but to whom you can refer to for other important decisions when the time comes.

It cannot be stressed enough that, in order to survive the caregiving process and avoid total burnout, you must set up support systems to help you. You do not have to do this alone. Help is available and the time you take to understand where it is, and how to access it, is crucial to your survival.

Surviving Caregiver Burnout

Caregiver burnout is a real condition and nothing to be taken lightly. It is described as "a state of physical, emotional, and mental exhaustion that may be accompanied by a change in attitude from positive and caring to negative and unconcerned." Burnout can occur for any number of reasons, but usually because the caregiver has tried to do more than they are physically, mentally, emotionally, or financially. Burnout symptoms include:

- Social withdrawal from friends, family, and loved ones;
- Loss of interest in activities previously enjoyed;
- A constant feeling of hopelessness or irritability and helplessness;
- Changes in weight, sleeplessness coupled with complete emotional and physical exhaustion;
- Frequent illness; and/or
- Feelings of depression that won't go away.

What Can Be Done to Avoid Burnout?

- You *must* have a support system in place (a plan follows).

- Set realistic goals and turn to others for relief with certain tasks.

- Be realistic about the illness that confronts you. Your role is not to heal, but to help make life manageable for your loved one.

- Set aside time for yourself. *This is not a luxury, but a necessity.*

- Talk to a professional if you feel your life is spinning out of control. You can't afford not to.

- Look into respite care services.

- Educate yourself. Take the time to research and learn. There is a plethora of information available.

- Do the basics. Eat right. Exercise. Get plenty of rest. Know when it's okay to turn off the phone and be quiet.

- Pamper yourself. Take a bath; a long shower; spend time in nature; tap into your own spirituality and ask for help.

- Accept your feelings of frustration and anger as normal. Better yet—celebrate them. They mean that you are *human!*

- Join a caregiver support group. Sharing your feelings with others in your same situation can be extremely helpful. Support groups help you manage stress, locate resources, and provide a venue to reduce feelings of frustration and isolation.

- Make time for activities you enjoy.

- Caregiving is rewarding, but there will be times when you will also feel anger, sadness, frustration, and grief. Try not to judge your feelings. They are neither good nor bad, but rather a normal part of being human.

Caregiving is hard work, filled with numerous demands. Sadly, many caregivers lose perspective about the importance of their role and feel guilty if they spend time on themselves. You cannot care for another person if you do not care for yourself. You must be kind to yourself and embrace the idea that your role as a caregiver is vital to our society. You are engaged in the ultimate service—giving of yourself to another person. Honor your role and honor yourself.

Setting Up Your Support System

Next to learning to set boundaries, nothing is as important as creating a support system for yourself. Life simply works better if we have people around us who we can rely on for emotional, spiritual, and intellectual support. When was the last time you asked for support? Really asked? The question becomes, when you are overwhelmed, do you ask for support? Do you reach out to your spouse or partner? Do you ask friends to help you? Or do you just keep it all inside? People don't know that you need help unless you ask. Most people want to help you.

As a caregiver, you simply cannot do this alone. Setting up your support team is not as easy as it sounds but, once you've established it, your life will be ever so much easier. I was once asked by a very wise woman if I had a good support team in place and, without really thinking, I said, "Yes, of course I do." And then I had to stop and really consider the answer to her question. And the truth was that I was a good support to many of my friends but, because I didn't ever ask for help and I certainly never appeared to need any help, I had friends, but not necessarily a support system. Another project for me. I had no idea how to go about this. Once again, I got quiet and tackled my fear—the fear of rejection. What if I asked and no one said, "Yes." What would I do then? There was only one way to find out. The steps I took actually worked and so I share them with you.

The first thing I did was sit at my computer to make a list of friends I trusted. Next to each name, I wrote something about the relationship I shared with this person. This is a key step, as not all of your friends can or will be willing to support you. Some of them are struggling too much in their own lives to give anything to you. Know the people you are asking and be clear about their limitations. I knew my family would be there for me, but I had never asked them for support, either. So I asked. They said yes. That was the easy part.

The next step was to ask others. How would I do this so it actually had meaning? I decided to write each person (all eight of them) an email. I laid out my situation, my frustrations, my challenges, and my limitations. I asked each one to support me in one specific way. These were not general requests for help. Be clear about your needs. And as I sent each email with great trepidation, I prayed that I would get a positive response. So each email went flying through cyberspace with a little spiritual help. And guess what? Each and every person answered me with a resounding, "Yes!" *Relief!* Now I had to put this system in place and actually work with my support team. The truth is that once you begin this process, life is never the same again. We work better in teams. Think about that for a second. People who work in vacuums are not easy to be around. Teamwork is what makes companies, large or small, successful. You are running a small business here and you need help. People want to help; they just need to be asked.

Use your support team as often as you need to. Sometimes it's just comforting to know there are people on whom you can call.

You can use the space below to do this exercise.

Notes:

Our Basic Human Needs

You know what you're supposed to do. You've read it 1000 times in every self-help book that has ever been written. There is no new information about basic human needs. I'm going to reiterate them and make them very plain and simple. You have to pay attention to your body. You have to listen to your soul and you have to be willing to be a little bit selfish. (Remember being selfish is not a bad thing.) These ideas become the same as a car alarm going off. No one pays attention to them anymore and yet, you look at the rate of stress-related illness like cancer: i.e. breast cancer (one in eight women) prostate (one in six men), obesity, depression, and you have to ask yourself, "What's causing this?" We're not just destined to get sick—but there is a lot of sickness in the world. There are a lot of things you can do to reduce the stress in your life and make it far more manageable.

Sleep

One of the first signs of caregiver burnout is a lack of sleep, and the inability to sleep even when you are exhausted. Managing your sleep is key to keeping yourself healthy. I hear women talking all the time about how they got only four or five hours sleep, almost as if they are really proud of this fact! It is not a contest to see who can walk around in a fog on the least amount of sleep! Numerous studies reveal that we need eight-to-nine hours a night in order to experience optimal mental and physical function. Now if you are in a caregiving situation, sleep is really challenging. I realized after Bob passed away that I hadn't really slept in over five years. The reason is that I was on call 24/7, 365 days a year and, when that condition is your life, you never really sleep soundly. The truth is that all of the crisis phone calls came in the middle of the night. My body learned to be on constant alert. I learned, however, how to manage this so that I wasn't a complete mess—sleep-deprived, yes, but not a complete mess.

I changed my sleeping habits. I went to bed earlier, turned off all the lights, did some quiet meditation before I slept, and gave my body permission to relax. I took some melatonin, wore an acupressure sleep patch, and drifted off to the most restful sleep I could. I never took sleeping aids because I couldn't risk being out of it if the phone rang, and, frankly, I don't take those kinds of medications. They leave me way too drowsy the next day.

You have to find your own way here, but understand that you must sleep. Your entire being depends on it. If you don't sleep, weight gain will be your new problem to overcome. Your skin and eyes will become dull and your brain will not operate properly. Take care of this and be serious about it. I have great respect for adults who take their sleep seriously.

Sleep Tips I've Learned Over the Years

Before you go to bed, practice some quiet meditation or at least deep breathing. You have to quiet your mind and breathing helps us do this.

If your brain is on overdrive, write your thoughts down and come back to them later. When the world gets quiet, our brains often wake up.

Try drinking a calming herbal tea before bed; chamomile works well.

Go to sleep at the same time every night.

Cut back on alcohol and eat dinner before seven p.m. No caffeine after three p.m.

If you can't fall asleep, try one of those white noise machines. They actually work.

The news can be very disrupting. Try watching it earlier in the evening.

You can try taking melatonin, valerian, or passionflower

about an hour before bedtime. (Melatonin works best for me and I play with the dosage depending on my need for rest.)

Allow yourself time to unwind and relax. Be gentle with yourself. You are under a tremendous amount of pressure and you need to figure out what actually works best for you. *But sleep!*

Your Diet Makes A Difference!

How are you nourishing your body? You already know that caregivng requires you to be on top of your daily game, and you need to be very aware of how you are fueling your body. It is not uncommon for caregivers to gain weight because suddenly, you have no personal time. Some caregivers lose weight but, again, that's not because they are trying to. You have to be committed to eating properly. This is not a book on nutrition, just a reminder that lack of food, too much junk food, and no supplementation will lead you to a place of sickness. You've got to be diligent. Take care of your body during this time in your life.

Exercise Matters!

Are you exercising? I know you don't have any time…but this comes back to boundaries. You don't have to become a marathon runner or a triathlete, but you must do something so that you can cope with your stress. You have to move your body. We know from the numerous studies done that exercise helps ward off depression but, better yet, it helps us feel good. It alleviates stress and helps prevent illness. You simply can't live a healthy life if you are lethargic. Yes, when we are exhausted it's easy to deny ourselves the opportunity to exercise, but it is probably the one thing you need to do most of all. Even if it's just taking a walk, moving helps the body work at optimum levels.

Find an exercise program that works for you. If it's a gym setting that you like, then go. If it's dancing, take a dance class. Yoga is great exercise and good for your mind and soul. If it's just walking in your neighborhood or at the beach, then do it. Schedule it and keep the appointment with yourself. I hike…that's my salvation. I take my dog or go by myself, listen to the sounds of nature or music in my ipod, and I'm gone for about an hour or so. I don't sacrifice myself for the sake of another. Do you call this selfish? I don't. It's an absolute MUST for me.

Don't Ignore Your Mental Health

When we ignore our mental stability our bodies scream at us. Many of us have been taught to stuff our feelings—to ignore them, to just "buck up." Well, when you do this, especially if you are in a traditional caregiving role, you are in trouble. I believe we need to embrace our negative feelings. They show up for a reason. They are yelling at you because you've ignored them. Honor your negative feelings just like you honor moments of joy. Sadness, anger, resentment, frustration, and even depression are all part and parcel of the caregiving experience. If you pay attention and tap into your feelings, the negative feelings will begin to fade and life will become more balanced. If you ignore them, they will continue to surface and wreak havoc with your well-being. Each morning when you arise, check in with yourself. How are you feeling? If it's joy—beautiful! Enjoy it. If it's depression or anger, give yourself a hug—a big hug, and ask for support. Allow yourself to feel the emotion for a day. Unless you are in real emotional trouble, chances are that these feelings will begin to dissipate. However, if you continue to feel rage, depression, or isolation, then seek help from a professional.

One common sign of caregiver burnout is the desire to be isolated from the rest of the world—family, friends, and social gatherings. This is different for each person, but common it is. If you feel yourself in this situation, I recommend that you get help.

If you have set up your support team, it's time to reach out and ask for support. I told you it was easier said than done.

Take a break, and that means hire some respite help if you can afford to, or arrange for one or two members from your support team to fill in for a few hours a week, so that you can really get away. Once you've made arrangements that you trust, (you can't relax until you trust that your time away is covered by a responsible person) then call a friend. Have a picnic. Go to the spa. Have lunch with someone who feeds your soul and who gives you positive energy. Rejuvenate yourself in any way you can. You must learn to listen to your soul and honor the feelings that are showing up for you. *You come first.*

Spirituality

I am a big believer in tapping into your spirituality. I couldn't have managed my caregiving years if I didn't surrender to something greater than myself. It was just too scary to think that the Universe wasn't speaking to me in some dynamic way. Spirituality is a daily practice for me. It's about staying in the present, living in gratitude, and not dwelling on past mistakes or future fears. I learned to pay attention to the signs along the way. I became more rooted in small moments of joy. I put my life in the hands of a greater power, because, even if I thought I knew better, I was often reminded that I was not really in control of the bigger things. I will not tell you how to tap into your spirituality. I can only suggest that believing in Something will help you move through your life with courage and grace and, at the end of the day, this, I believe, is what we all are hoping for.

One of the ways I learned to manage my stress and connect more with my own spirituality was through meditation. In the beginning it felt awkward, but as I practiced and listened to tapes, I became much calmer and serenity began to set in. If you are not familiar with this age-old practice, you might want to give meditation a try.

Life is a journey and it's paved with strife and turmoil and even disaster, but it's also filled with opportunity, fiery sunsets, joy, laughter, and abundance, and it's really our choice. It's about finding our own personal *yes* and really waking up each day and choosing to be the best that we can.

You might be someone who hasn't experienced any strife along the way, and crisis hasn't graced your doorstep, but I want you to remember that in a moment your life can change. So will you be prepared and have your personal caring house in order? A part of me wishes I had done this work earlier, but the reality is that it took Bob, my former father-in-law, on a Sunday night to change the Cindy who I had become so familiar with.

I now wake up every day and have the same dialogue with myself. What will I be called upon to do today? How will I handle it? And I know that some days will be great, some days not so good, and some just okay. But we choose how we walk through this life. There are no do-overs. This is all we get and so the choice is ours. Celebrate your life. Celebrate the life you have been asked to care for. You have taken on the most beautiful of all roles and that is to care for another.

William Shakespeare said, "It is one of the most beautiful compensations of this life that no man can sincerely try to help another without helping himself."

## PART III

Forms and Resources

This section is designed to assist you in getting organized. Use the forms as you wish, but make sure you keep the original and make copies. A CD of all the forms is included at the end of the guide. As you travel along the caregiving journey, you will be amazed at the amount of paperwork that you need to complete on a monthly and annual basis. Much of it is repetitive, but needs to be done routinely. Keeping copious records will expedite the process and make your life more manageable. Chances are there are more forms than you will need; but just in case, they're here for your comfort and organization.

Important Phone Numbers

In Case of Emergency   **Call 911**
Emergency Hospital   _____
Local Police Station   _____
Local Fire Dept   _____

Doctor's Phone Numbers
Primary Care Physician   _____
Cardiologist   _____
Neurologist   _____
Ophthalmologist   _____
Pharmacologist   _____
Psychiatrist/Psychologist   _____
Podiatrist   _____
Pulmonary Specialist   _____
Urologist   _____
Dentist   _____
Personal Trainer   _____
Physical Therapist   _____
Social Worker   _____

Service Numbers
Appliance Repair   _____
Cable Repair   _____
Car Repair   _____
Country Club Numbers   _____
Electrician

Handyman   _____

Gardener   _____

Pharmacy   _____

Phone Repair   _____

Plumber   _____

Pool and Spa   _____

Security System   _____

Veterinarian   _____

Professional Consultants

Accountant   _____

Attorney   _____

Financial Advisor   _____

Insurance Agent   _____

Personal Banker   _____

Realtor   _____

Family Phone Numbers

Caregiver's Phone Numbers

Housekeeper   _____

Senior Information Sheet

Name:_____

Address:_____

_____

Phone Number: _____

Cell : _____

Date of Birth:_____

Vital Medical Information: _____

_____

_____

_____

_____

_____

_____

_____

_____

Location of nearest hospital _____

_____

Name of Hospital: _____

Address:_____

_____

Phone: _____

Directions from home:

Senior's History, Hobbies, and Interests

This page is perhaps the most important one in the care guide as it will educate others about your loved one's personal history.

The Senior's Personal History

Born: _____

Grew Up: _____

Moved To: _____

Education: _____

Member of the Military: ____yes ____no

Branch: _____

Served in a War: ____yes _____no

Which War? _____

Married: _____

Number of Children: _____

Professions: _____

_____

_____

_____

Special Talents: _____

_____

_____

Hobbies:_____

_____

_____

Athletic Interests: _____

_____

_____

Special Interests:_____

_____

_____

Favorite Movies:_____

_____

_____

Favorite Music:_____

_____

_____

Religious Practices: _____

_____

_____

Special Accomplishments: _____

_____

_____

Emergency Contacts

Name:_____

Relationship: _____

Phones: Home: _____

Work: _____   Cell: _____

Email: _____

Name:_____

Relationship: _____

Phones: Home: _____

Work: _____   Cell: _____

Email: _____

Name:_____

Relationship: _____

Phones: Home: _____

Work: _____   Cell: _____

Email: _____

Insurance Information

Record all insurance information here. *Do not attach originals.*

Primary Health Insurance Carrier

Name of Company: _____

Patient's ID #: _____

Group Number: _____

Phone Number of Carrier: _____

Secondary Health Insurance Carrier

Name of Company: _____

_____

Patient's ID #: _____

Group Number: _____

Phone Number of Carrier: _____

Primary Care Physician Information

You do not need to complete this form for all the doctors; however, this is great information to have at your fingertips especially when an emergency arises.

Doctor's Name:_____

Group Name (if affiliated): _____

Address:_____

_____

Phone Number: _____

Fax Number: _____

Email: _____

Receptionist's Name: _____

Nurse's Name: _____

Patient's Blood Type: _____

Known Medication/Drug Allergies:

Known Food Allergies:

Medication Information Sheets

It is a well-known fact that many seniors take up to thirty medications daily! Yes, it's shocking, but it is the way of our world and keeping track of these medications can be a full-time job in and of itself. (Do you understand now why you don't want an untrained caregiver to be responsible for prescription disbursement?) When all of these medications begin interacting with one another, it becomes very challenging to manage it all. Maintaining an organized list of all medications, and the doctors who have prescribed them, will give your primary care physician a leg up on managing this aspect of the senior's life. Do not take this step lightly as all medications have side effects and if not administered correctly, can be life-threatening.

Consider purchasing a medication dispenser box. I recommend using a weekly dispenser box, as it is less confusing for the senior. It's highly possible that you will need to purchase two of them—one for morning medications and one for evening. Label each box clearly so there is no confusion. Most of these prescriptions need to be taken at different times of the day. *You* will be responsible for putting the medications in the daily boxes. You should also be prepared to call on a daily basis and make sure that the medications have been taken. Check when you visit to see that this has been done.

In addition, a *Master Prescription Sheet* is a good idea when trying to keep track of all the different medications. Often a visit to the doctor will involve a new medication or the changing of one for another. Be sure to keep this sheet updated. This record keeping is extremely helpful when an emergency happens, as you will be required to inform paramedics or doctors at the emergency hospital of all medications being taken. In a time of crisis it's almost impossible to remember and the prescription record is invaluable.

Unless you want to re-do this sheet frequently (and you don't) I recommend you write it in pencil or keep it in a computer file that is easy to update and print out new copies as needed. Another good tip is to develop a trusting relationship with the pharmacist if possible. Doctors are short on time and relationships with pharmacists and nurses can be very helpful.

Medication Information

Name of Medication: _____

Prescribing doctor: _____

Date medication prescribed: _____

Reason for prescription: _____

_____

Dosage: _____

# of times taken per day _____

Side effects experienced: _____

_____

Date medication is discontinued: _____

Reason for discontinuing: _____

_____

Name of Medication: _____

Prescribing doctor: _____

Date medication prescribed: _____

Reason for prescription: _____

_____

Dosage: _____

# of times taken per day _____

Side effects experienced: _____

_____

Date medication is discontinued: _____

Reason for discontinuing: _____

_____

Name of Medication: _____

Prescribing doctor: _____

Date medication prescribed: _____

Reason for prescription: _____

_____

Dosage: _____

# of times taken per day _____

Side effects experienced: _____

_____

Date medication is discontinued: _____

Reason for discontinuing: _____

_____

Vitamins, Herbs, and Supplements

Vitamins, herbs, and supplements, considered natural, often interfere with the efficacy of prescription medications. This does not mean that they need to be discontinued, but you do need to keep a current list of what is being taken and ask the doctor if any of them interfere with prescription medications. (Do not trust what you are told at the local supplement store. These people are not trained in pharmacology.)

Name:_____

Brand:_____

Dosage: _____

# of times taken per day _____

Reason for taking: _____

_____

Side effects (if any): _____

_____

Reason for discontinuing: _____

_____

Name:_____

Brand:_____

Dosage: _____

# of times taken per day _____

Reason for taking: _____

_____

Side effects (if any): _____

_____

Reason for discontinuing: _____

_____

Name:_____

Brand:_____

Dosage: _____

# of times taken per day _____

Reason for taking: _____

_____

Side effects (if any): _____

_____

Reason for discontinuing: _____

_____

Name:_____

Brand:_____

Dosage: _____

# of times taken per day _____

Reason for taking: _____

_____

Side effects (if any): _____

_____

Reason for discontinuing: _____

_____

Pharmacy Information

I cannot stress enough the importance of dealing with one pharmacy. Many offer free delivery if you do all of your business with them, and you will remember that developing a relationship with the pharmacist can be extremely helpful when you are managing multiple prescriptions from a different doctors.

Name of Primary Pharmacy: _____

_____

Contact Person:_____

Address:_____

_____

Phone Number: _____

Fax Number: _____

Email: _____

Website: _____

Name of Secondary Pharmacy:_____

_____

Contact Person:_____

Address:_____

_____

Phone Number: _____

Fax Number: _____

Email: _____

Website: _____

Notes:

Daily Monitoring

If you have outside help in the house, then you must insist on daily records. Make it a part of the job description. If anyone balks at this idea—move on. Any caregiver or medical professional should do this task willingly. If done properly, it means they are covered in the event that things go wrong. Details matter.

Ask the caregiver to be as precise as possible, as this is your way of knowing exactly what is being done in the home when you are not present. Be sure that the caregiver makes note of unusual phone calls or strangers coming to the door. If there are outings, make sure they are recorded. If, by some chance, the senior trips and falls, even if there is no apparent injury, then it must be recorded. Everything and anything. The more detail the better. Ask each caregiver to sign or initial next to the entry and request clear handwriting.

I recommend that you reproduce these on a monthly basis just to save time. Keep them in a large binder and section them off by month. Should you ever need to refer to them, you will have the senior/patient's daily history at your fingertips. Consider the daily monitoring sheets your personal view of your loved one's daily activities. Be sure you check them when you arrive at the house to visit. Even if you don't read them word for word, the hired caregiver must see that you are paying attention to detail. If you are the caregiver, it's a way of accounting for your daily activities and it provides important information for the medical team. Each month remove the old ones and print out a new batch of sheets.

Daily Monitoring Sheets

Patient: _____

Date: _____

Completed by _____

6:00am

7:00am

8:00am

9:00am

10:00am

11:00am

Noon

1:00pm

2:00pm

3:00pm

4:00pm

5:00pm

6:00pm

7:00pm

8:00pm

9:00pm

10:00pm

Midnight

1:00am

2:00am

3:00am

4:00am

5:00am

Additional Notes or Observations:

Personal Care Requirements

Personal Hygiene

Bath: _____

Shampoo:_____

Oral Care: _____

Post Toilet Care: _____

Skin Care: _____

Fluids

Preferences: _____

Restricted: _____

Elimination

Continent? _____

Pads? _____

Constipation controlled with:_____

Diarrhea controlled with: _____

Activity

Walking:_____

Exercise: _____

Assistance needed? _____

Mobility devices used:_____

Fall precautions: _____

Sensory Status

Vision: _____

Hearing:_____

New Observations:

Caregiver Task List

Housekeeping Responsibilities

Activity	Frequency		
	Daily	Weekly	Other
Make Bed			
Change Linens			
Clean Kitchen			
Wash Dishes			
Clean Bathroom			
Dust Furniture			
Vacuum			
Laundry			
Groceries			

Personal Care Responsibilities

Activity	Frequency		
Bathing			
Wash Hair			
Toileting			
Exercising			
Walking			
Meal Prep			

Notes:

Current Health Issues

I am not a big believer in self-diagnosis, but many seniors and caregivers engage in this activity. Seniors have a whole host of medical issues to manage. Some are serious and some are just life's little obstacles to overcome, and some seniors are good at creating issues when they feel the need for attention. If a problem is lingering, getting worse, or becomes persistent, call the doctor immediately. We are not trained physicians and you cannot ignore medical issues that present and do not subside or go away.

I once cared for a woman who lived alone and her children seldom came to visit. She was very "with it" and her favorite thing to do when she was feeling lonely, or woke up with an ailment, was to self-diagnose and call the paramedics to take her to the emergency hospital. She hated the hospital, but her need for attention was more powerful than the hospital experience.

As Bob's dementia became worse, he began remembering past injuries. I received a call one day that his shoulder was really bothering him and that he couldn't move it. I had no idea how this could have happened as he had nurses caring for him around the clock. When I arrived, he told me about his diving accident! *Diving accident?* I thought. After several minutes of him wincing in excruciating pain, he told me about an accident that he had when he was in high school! I knew that dementia was in control. He screamed, wouldn't let anyone touch him and finally I called the doctor. Yes, we went for a "dementia x-ray" because he could and it was the only thing that would calm him down.

I share these two stories with you because it exemplifies the power of the mind. Then again, there are cases when a senior will have serious digestive problems and have diarrhea or constipation for days (often as a side effect of medications) and nothing will be said about this, all the while, the senior is become dehydrated or bloated and uncomfortable. Conditions like this can be very serious and definitely require a doctor's visit.

Pay attention to what is going on. Call the doctor and ask for advice. If you have forged a relationship here, the doctor's office will be most accommodating. However, you should definitely keep track of any changes in health and well-being.

Current Health Issues

New medical issue:

How long has problem existed?_____

Describe the symptoms:

Any fever? _____yes _____no _____how high?

Contacted doctor: _____yes _____no _____date

Doctor's name: _____

Outcome:

Eyeglass Information

Optometrist: _____

Address:_____

_____

Phone: _____

Fax: _____

Email: _____

# of Annual Appointments Needed _____

Dentist Information

Dentist:_____

Address:_____

_____

Phone: _____

Fax: _____

Email: _____

# of Annual Appointments Needed _____

Planning for Emergencies

You need to take this seriously. Having the necessary procedures in place in case of an emergency is well worth your time and effort. Seniors became extremely frightened in emergencies. They fear the worst and trust you to take care of them. Make plans to give them peace of mind.

If you have caregivers in the home, you should have an emergency exit route written down so there is no confusion. Figure out the easiest path to exit the house in case of a natural disaster, fire, etc. Include your plan in this manual.

Emergency Items Needed

- Flashlight with extra batteries
- Cell phone with charger
- Water (one gallon of water per person per day for at least three days)
- Food (non-perishable food, enough for three days)
- Battery-powered radio
- Extra clothing and undergarments (if needed)
- First Aid Kit
- Loud whistle to signal for help
- Dust mask (seniors are very sensitive to dust)
- Plastic sheeting and duct tape for shelter
- Moist towelettes, garbage bags, and plastic ties for sanitation
- Wrench or pliers to turn off utilities
- Can opener

Additional Items

- Prescription medications and glasses
- Pet food and extra water if you have a pet (don't forget a leash)
- Important family documents such as copies of insurance policies, identification, and bank account records kept in a waterproof, portable container
- Cash or traveler's checks and change
- Sleeping bag or warm blanket for each person. Consider additional bedding if you live in a cold climate.
- Complete change of clothing including a long-sleeved shirt, long pants, and sturdy shoes. Consider additional clothing if you live in a cold climate.
- Household chlorine bleach and medicine dropper (When diluted nine parts water to one part bleach, bleach can be used as a disinfectant. Or in an emergency, you can use it to treat water by using sixteen drops of regular household liquid bleach per gallon of water. Do not use scented, color safe, or bleaches with added cleaners.)
- Matches in a waterproof container
- Mess kits, paper cups, plates and plastic utensils, paper towels
- Paper and pencil

Hospital Preparedness

Hospitals are scary places and your best defense to help offset the fear is to bring some items from home that help the senior feel more comfortable. Also, by having this bag packed in advance, you are always prepared.

Keep in Bag at all Times

- Pajamas (a few pairs)
- Robe/slippers
- Underwear
- Socks
- Cozy soft blanket for chilly hospital rooms
- Toothbrush and toothpaste
- Deodorant
- Facecloths
- Face and body lotion
- Comb/Brush
- Extra pair of eyeglasses
- Copy of Power of Attorney, Medical Directive, and insurance forms

Add to Bag When Leaving

- Bring the manual with all information.
- Leave medications at home, as you can't use them in the hospital.
- Cell phone and charger
- Wallet/purse

- Address book
- Dentures or hearing aids

If the senior is going to be in the hospital for a longer stay, it's nice to bring pillows from home and perhaps a quilt or blanket that is special. Family photos also make a difference.

Diet and Nutrition

This is a particularly challenging topic. Seniors are often on restricted diets. They may have developed sensitivities to foods or they might have allergies or dietary restrictions due to religious beliefs. They may have physical problems, which make eating a challenge. Many seniors have a problem chewing food due to missing teeth or dentures.

Some are at risk of aspiration because of swallowing difficulties. Over time some foods become more difficult to digest and, thus, there are more frequent bouts with constipation or diarrhea. This is serious because dehydration and edema are common and serious problems for seniors. Most seniors suffer from dehydration. Finding a way to convince them that they need to drink fluids (water, Gatorade) and not soda is really important for their overall health and wellness.

Then there is the challenge of loss of appetite. As we age, our taste buds lose their sensitivity and, as a result, many seniors lose their appetite. Food just doesn't taste good. Have you ever noticed that most seniors relish carbohydrates, sugar, and salt? There's a reason for this. Foods rich in sugar or salt have more flavor and provide instant satisfaction. The fact of the matter is that seniors, for the most part, don't really care what's good for them. They eat to stay alive and they want what they want. Of course, you have to control this in some way, but I also believe that quality of life is important. You cannot be the food police all the time at every meal.

Negotiation usually works well. Offer a choice of foods. Let the senior decide. Does it really matter what one eats for breakfast or dinner? Your concern is nutrition. You can puree fruit into a smoothie, but it doesn't matter if it's at breakfast or dinner. When a senior's health is declining, I am more concerned about moments of grace, dignity, and happiness, than whether or not all nutrients are eaten on a daily basis. (This is just a personal feeling after dealing with this subject for years.) Try to avoid having arguments over food. Be flexible and work together for the greater good of the senior in question.

The following sheet is for outside caregivers who might be cooking or shopping in your absence. It serves as an informational guideline.

Diet and Nutrition Information

Food Preferences

Breakfast

Lunch

Snacks

Dinner

Least favorite foods—list foods here that you know will never be consumed:

Food sensitivities—llist any foods that create digestive or swallowing issues:

Food allergies—list any foods that must be eliminated from the diet:

Food Restrictions due to health-related medical conditions or for religious beliefs:

Safety First!

You must, must, must make the home safe. What might look like a normal house to you can literally be a death trap. As we age, our physical and mental capabilities decline, thus making what was once a friendly home full of trinkets and years of accumulation now becomes a place that requires cautious maneuvering.

Night vision is not what it used to be. Stability and balance change. Walking up and down stairs becomes a major event. Finding items in drawers that once were familiar, is now a chore. Cooking food is a challenge. Remembering to turn off the stove or oven is worrisome. When a senior knows that he/she is failing, it becomes easier to stay in one room and not venture out. You must make the house safe and you can involve your loved one in this process. I have created a very detailed scavenger hunt game for your use in elder-proofing the home. This is a great exercise to do as a family. Involve the senior in the process and if there are grandchildren around, ask them to participate. Now it becomes a family activity.

The Elder-Proof-Your-Home Scavenger Hunt

Having fun while doing mundane chores is a great way to approach life. When your elderly loved ones want to live independently in their home, there are safety precautions you must take. Have a good time with this project and involve your loved one(s). This is a *Safety Scavenger Hunt!* Embark on this project together, follow the directions, and you will have created a safe and comfortable environment together.

Danger zone: Look for the following dangerous items and situations and clean them up first.

Throw rugs—One in every three seniors over the age of sixty-five will fall this year. Throw rugs are a huge problem as many seniors trip over them. *Remove all throw rugs.*

Glass tabletops—Glass is extremely hazardous regarding a fall or even bumping into corners. Replace with safe tabletops.

Heavy objects in high places—The last thing you want is for heavy objects to fall on your loved one's head! Clean out shelves and store heavy items properly in lower cabinets.

Fragile items—Take them off tabletops or secure them with Quake Wax (used in museums and available at hardware stores).

Toxic cleaning supplies—Get rid of these items and replace with non-toxic "green" cleaning supplies. Store in one place so as to avoid confusion.

Furniture and "stuff" obstructions—Move anything that is in the way of a clear walking path. Clean up these areas, so tripping doesn't occur. (What seems like a simple maneuver to you is often a hazard to a senior with balance issues.)

Electrical cords—Keep all electrical cords and cables out of the way. They present a major hazard in the home.

Interior door locks—Change out interior locking door mechanisms with doorknobs that do not lock or simply cover them with plastic covers (available in baby stores). You can also purchase a door plate, which makes it impossible to lock the door (very inexpensive and worth it).

Label kitchen cupboards, cabinets, **bathroom** drawers, and **dresser** drawers with the contents of each.

Medicine cabinet—Every bathroom has one and most haven't been cleaned out for years. Take precautions to clean the cabinet and get rid of any toxic medicine or expired medications. Its purpose now is to contain items like Band-Aids, toothpaste, or any other item that will not hurt your loved one.

Emergency equipment—You need to have the proper emergency equipment in place, and it is essential that your loved one be clear about where these items are located.
First aid kit—Bathroom and kitchen

Fire extinguisher—Kitchen

Smoke alarms—Place them throughout the house. (They save lives!)

Flashlights—Wall-mounted flashlights need to be placed in obvious places. You cannot have too many of these: kitchen, laundry room, bathrooms, and one on either side of the bed for quick access.

Nightlights—Any pathway that will require entry when it's dark needs to be illuminated with nightlights. You can't have too many.

Check periodically and see if your loved one remembers where these items are located. Never move anything important without alerting your loved one.

Emergency information—This is very important. Create a list in large font that has all necessary emergency numbers. Organize it by category. 911 is first. Then add family members, neighbors, doctors, and any other numbers that might be needed. Remember, large font! Place a list next to every phone and secure it to a table or wall for easy access.

It is also absolutely necessary that you keep a list of emergency numbers, medications, any allergies, and doctor's numbers on an information sheet or card in a purse or wallet.

You should have a copy of this list, too, and you might consider providing the same list to a neighbor as well as the person designated to be your back-up.

Now Let's Take it Room by Room!

Check when task is completed.

Kitchen—One of the most dangerous rooms in the house. You have to alter your thinking to ensure proper safety. You cannot remove all the hazards, but with some modifications, you can make the kitchen a must less hazardous room.

_____Remove any and all throw rugs.

_____Change towel bars, wooden, metal, or ceramic, and replace with sturdy grab bars. Think about falling. If your loved one loses his/her balance the first thing reached for is a towel bar. They are not meant to support human weight. Grab bars can and often do save lives.

_____Move hard-to-reach objects that are frequently used to lower shelves.

_____Install a smoke alarm and change the batteries every six months. (Good idea to do it when daylight savings begins and when it ends.)

_____Purchase a first aid kit for the kitchen and have it easily accessible.

_____Keep frequently used products such as dishwashing soap, sponges, and paper towels in an easy-to-reach location.

_____NO PAPER PRODUCTS NEAR THE STOVE!

_____Toxic products—out of reach and out of sight. Replace with green/non-toxic cleaning supplies.

_____If your loved one has a difficult time feeling the push buttons on the microwave, add Velcro buttons on top of the existing buttons. Green for start and red for stop. (As we age, the feeling in our fingertips becomes less sensitive. This trick helps.)

_____If you must…purchase a one-step safety stool that has supports on both sides and in the front, but only if your loved can handle this task. Do a test and see.

_____If you are worried about the stove, purchase stove knob covers.

Bedroom—Seniors often spend a good portion of their day in the bedroom. It is critical that this room be the most comfortable and extremely safe.

_____Remove all throw rugs. If this is impossible, then secure them with reflective tape.

_____Remove all sharp, heavy, fragile, or unbalanced items from surfaces, shelves, and tabletops. If there are items that are special then secure them with Quake Wax, used in museums and very strong.

_____Label dresser drawers and keep clothing in the proper place. Organize clothes in closet for easy access.

_____No candles. Install at least two wall-mounted flashlights in the bedroom. Nightlights are necessary as well. Make sure nothing is blocking a walkway.

_____It's a good idea to have a reacher to avoid over-reaching, which, again, can cause falls.

_____Keep books, cards, favorite music, and DVDs in the room where the most time is spent. Make the investment in your loved one's "favorites."

_____Comfortable chair. This might be a lift chair or any chair that is a favorite and is placed near good light with easy access.

_____Magnifying glass. Purchase several large magnifying glasses and keep them handy. Nothing fancy, just functional.

_____Doorknobs. Make sure doorknobs can never be locked from the inside. You can change them or purchase doorknob covers.

_____Install a smoke alarm and change batteries every six months.

Bathroom—This is another hazardous area unless you take precautions to make it a safety zone.

_____GRAB BARS, GRAB BARS, GRAB BARS. You can't have too many of them. Stand in the bathroom and figure out where or how a fall might occur and then install a bar to offer support. Replace all towel bars with grab bars.

_____Shower seat. This can make all the difference in having a pleasant showering experience vs. one that is really challenging. Hot water is often fatiguing for the elderly or infirmed and it's easy to lose one's balance when relaxed.

_____Remove all throw rugs.

_____Purchase an anti-slip treatment for placement in the tub or shower. For the obvious reason, you need to purchase an anti-slip mat.

_____Pill container. You need this in order to organize medications. Purchase a large one that's easy to see and one that has easy access. (Depending upon the situation, you might need to call and remind your loved one to take medications. Check on this regularly to make sure the meds are being taken appropriately.)

_____Remove all sharp, fragile, or heavy objects like in the rest of the house.

_____Equip the bathroom with a wall-mounted flashlight.

_____Remove all toxic products.

_____Label all drawers for easy recognition.

_____Keep frequently used supplies in an easy-to-reach location: Washcloths, soap, toothbrush, toothpaste (use the old-fashioned tube), comb, brush, etc.

Living Room/Family Room/Den—Whatever you call it, this room presents hazards. Most elderly people don't choose to spend a lot of time in this room, but don't ignore the reality that it presents hazards. Make it safe.

_____Remove all throw rugs. Tripping leads to falling and falling leads to broken bones or head injuries.

_____Unstable tables should be removed or stabilized. Beware of glass tabletops.

_____Footstools can also lead to falls. Remove them entirely or place them out of walkways.

_____Remove sharp objects from tables, bookshelves, or any high surface.

_____Fragile objects should be stored in a safe place or moved to a safe location.

_____Remove heavy objects that might fall and cause injury.

_____Secure table lamps and fragile items with Quake Wax.

_____Remove all candles and have a flashlight handy.

_____If there are steps leading (even one or two) to the living room, add a handrail.

Halls, Doorways, and Stairs—These areas are often ignored and the ones where the most accidents occur, usually because they are not well lit.

_____Fix the lighting. You might have to have motion lights installed, but it's worth every penny that you spend on an electrician.

_____Again, remove all throw rugs.

_____You can purchase small threshold ramps to minimize accidents or add reflective tape to the stairs to minimize danger.

_____Make sure that all handrails are secure.

Garage and Basement—A real danger zone especially since these are the areas where clutter accumulates. I always recommend that your elderly loved one stay out of these places. It's easy to get someone in the family, a neighbor, or a friend to retrieve whatever is needed.

_____Good lighting is a must.

_____Remove all rakes, brooms, shovels, and any gardening tools. They are hazardous items and should be safely stored in some kind of cupboard or shed.

_____Consider boxing the clutter and making a donation to charity or storing on shelves. Whatever you do, remove the clutter from these areas.

The Changing Seasons –As much as most of us welcome seasonal changes, for seniors, weather is often a hazard. Snow shoveling is *not* a job for seniors. Cleaning rain gutters: *not* a job for seniors. Pruning roses: *not* a job for seniors. Raking leaves: *not* a job for seniors. You get the picture. Minimize the risk and hire someone to do these jobs.

Congratulations, you've now created a home that is safe, and hazard-free. However, you must understand that there is always a risk. I've linked a company that I trust to provide you with reputable and affordable products on my website. Look in the resources section of this manual for my recommendations.

The Family Pet

The human-animal bond is a powerful one, and studies have shown that animals can have a beneficial effect on human health and emotional well-being. More and more service animals are being brought into hospitals and nursing homes to provide comfort and companionship. The connection is instant and there are numerous stories espousing the magic that exists between humans and animals.

I am a huge proponent of bringing an animal into the home of your loved one, providing the animal receives the proper care. Beautiful bonds between seniors or anyone who is handicapped and animals have been documented, and many who suffer from depression can find love and comfort from having a pet. But pet care takes time and is another responsibility. Think carefully about this decision.

If a pet is already living in your loved one's home, then you really have no other choice except to make sure that proper care is provided. It is possible that your loved one has become lax in this area and you may need to take a trip to the veterinarian just to make certain that everything is okay. If you are in a position to hire outside help to walk or run a dog or to have someone come in and feed the senior's pet, this is one way to help minimize your responsibility and gives everyone peace of mind. If you can, it's also a nice idea to consider having a mobile groomer come every couple of months. You don't want to be bringing extra dirt and germs into the house, so this really alleviates a lot of extra labor for you.

Animals provide a huge amount of companionship and the joy that is brought to the home is often worth the extra investment in time and money.

Make sure you keep a current photo of the animal in this notebook in case it gets out.

Family Pet Information

Pet's Name: _____

Date of Birth: _____

Species: _____

Diet: _____

Number of Feedings per Day: _____

Number of Walks per Day (if applicable): _____

Allergies or Special Conditions: _____

_____

Veterinarian Information

Name of Doctor: _____

Name of Group: _____

Address: _____

_____

Phone Number: _____

Fax Number: _____

Email: _____

Alternate doctor in case primary doctor is unavailable:

_____

Legal and Financial Information

I am not an attorney nor am I an accountant, and I do not profess to be either one. Most families have professionals who have been dealing with family matters for years. However, no manual would be complete without addressing some of the issues that arise as seniors journey through the aging process. Keeping all of the senior's information in one place makes the process much easier.

If you are taking over the personal legal and financial affairs for the senior, there are many matters that you must handle. The Power of Attorney decisions were previously dealt with in this manual.(Forms are not included in the care guide as they vary from state to state.) Do not be surprised if legal, financial, and insurance matters are unorganized and in chaos. A few phone calls and meetings will straighten everything out.

Take your time as you tackle this component of the senior's life and use the forms provided to help you get organized and keep all vital information in one place.

A Word of Caution

Do not keep sensitive documents or information in this binder. You should have a special place designated for these types of documents or information. Simply indicate where the information is located so that the person responsible for keeping track of these documents knows how to access it. Keep all legal documents in one place. Consider the following:

- Birth Certificate
- Citizenship Papers (if applicable)
- Death Certificate (of spouse)
- Driver's License
- Marriage License
- Military Discharge Papers
- Mortgage Information
- Passport
- Power of Attorney—Finances
- Power of Attorney—Healthcare
- Property Deed
- Social Security Card
- Tax Information
- Title to Car

Legal and Financial Professionals

Attorney

Name:_____

Law Firm: _____

Secretary/Assistant's Name: _____

Address:_____

_____

Phone: _____

Fax: _____

Email: _____

Legal matters handled by this attorney: _____

_____

_____

Attorney

Name:_____

Law Firm: _____

Secretary/Assistant's Name: _____

Address:_____

_____

Phone: _____

Fax: _____

Email: _____

Legal matters handled by this attorney: _____

_____

_____

Accountant/CPA

Name:_____

Company: _____

Secretary/Assistant's Name: _____

Address:_____

_____

Phone: _____

Fax: _____

Email: _____

Financial Advisor

Name:_____

Company: _____

Secretary/Assistant's Name: _____

Address:_____

Phone: _____

Fax: _____

Email: _____

Account Numbers and Information:

Insurance Broker

Name:_____

Company: _____

Secretary/Assistant's Name: _____

Address:_____

_____

Phone: _____

Fax: _____

Email: _____

Account Numbers and Information:

Power of Attorney (Financial)

Name:_____

Relationship to senior:_____

Address:_____

Phone: _____

Fax: _____

Email: _____

Durable Power of Attorney for Health

Name:_____

Relationship to senior:_____

Address:_____

_____

Phone: _____

Fax: _____

Email: _____

Financial Institutions

Name of Bank/Financial Institution: _____

_____

Banker's Name (if any): _____

Address:_____

Phone: _____

Fax: _____

Web site:_____

Account Information

Checking Account Number:_____

Password/Pin: _____

Password Hint: _____

_____

Savings Account Number: _____

Password/Pin: _____

Password Hint:_____

_____

CD Information _____

_____

Safety Deposit Box Number: _____

Location of Keys: _____

Person responsible for Keys: _____

Credit Card Information

Credit Card: Type of Card _____

Account #: _____

Password/Pin: _____

Password Hint: _____

_____

Customer Service Information

Phone: _____

Fax: _____

Address:_____

_____

Credit Card: Type of Card _____

Account #: _____

Password/Pin: _____

Password Hint: _____

_____

Customer Service Information

Phone: _____

Fax: _____

Address:_____

_____

Credit Card: Type of Card _____

Account #: _____

Password/Pin: _____

Password Hint: _____

_____

Customer Service Information

Phone: _____

Fax: _____

Address:_____

_____

Insurance

Our lives are sometimes run by the insurance premiums and policies that we keep for times of emergencies. Your life will be much easier to manage if you keep all insurance information in one place—**here**. Some families have up to ten different insurance policies all covering different aspects of their lives. In my experience most seniors have different insurance agents for different policies. Do not hesitate to reach out to the insurance brokers for assistance in understanding your loved one's policy. Personally I think insurance policies are like reading Greek. The senior has probably been paying premiums for years, so now is the time to ask for help in repayment for all the money paid.

Insurance Information

Auto Insurance: First Auto

Name of Company: _____

Agent's Name: _____

Address:_____

_____

Phone: _____

Fax: _____

Email: _____

Account #: _____

Make: _____ Model: _____

Year: _____ Color: _____

Location of Policy: _____

Auto Insurance: Second Auto

Name of Company: _____

Agent's Name: _____

Address:_____

_____

Phone: _____

Fax: _____

Email: _____

Account #: _____

Make: _____ Model: _____

Year: _____ Color: _____

Location of Policy: _____

Homeowner's Insurance

Name of Company: _____

Agent's Name: _____

Address: _____

_____

Phone: _____

Fax: _____

Email: _____

Account #: _____

Location of Policy: _____

_____

Liability Insurance

Name of Company: _____

Agent's Name: _____

Address:_____

_____

Phone: _____

Fax: _____

Email: _____

Account #: _____

Location of Policy: _____

_____

Long-Term Care Insurance

Name of Company: _____

Agent's Name: _____

Address:_____

_____

Phone: _____

Fax: _____

Email: _____

Account #: _____

Location of Policy: _____

_____

Life Insurance

Name of Company: _____

Agent's Name: _____

Address:_____

_____

Phone: _____

Fax: _____

Email: _____

Account #: _____

Amount of Benefit:_____

Location of Policy: _____

_____

Other Insurance

Name of Company: _____

Agent's Name: _____

Address:_____

_____

Phone: _____

Fax: _____

Email: _____

Account #: _____

Location of Policy: _____

_____

Other Insurance

Name of Company: _____

Agent's Name: _____

Address:_____

_____

Phone: _____

Fax: _____

Email: _____

Account #: _____

Location of Policy: _____

_____

Personal Property—Vehicles

Vehicle Information—Vehicle 1

Make and Model: _____

Date of Purchase/Loan: _____

Date Sold/Purchaser: _____

Location of Pink Slip:_____

Contact Person:_____

Registration:

Make/Model/Year _____

Renewal Due: _____

Vehicle Information—Vehicle 2

Make and Model: _____

Date of Purchase/Loan: _____

Date Sold/Purchaser: _____

Location of Pink Slip:_____

Contact Person:_____

Registration:

Make/Model/Year _____

Renewal Due: _____

Personal Property—Valuables

Jewelry

Description: _____

_____

Location: _____

Appraisal: _____ yes _____ no

Where kept? _____

To be given to whom: _____

Description: _____

_____

Location: _____

Appraisal: _____ yes _____ no

Where kept? _____

To be given to whom: _____

Description: _____

_____

Location: _____

Appraisal: _____yes _____ no

Where kept? _____

To be given to whom: _____

Description: _____

_____

Location: _____

Appraisal: _____yes _____ no

Where kept? _____

To be given to whom: _____

Description: _____

_____

Location: _____

Appraisal: _____yes _____ no

Where kept? _____

To be given to whom: _____

Furniture and Art

Description:_____

_____

Location: _____

Appraisal: _____yes _____ no

Where kept? _____

To be given to whom: _____

Description:_____

_____

Location: _____

Appraisal: _____yes _____ no

Where kept? _____

To be given to whom: _____

Description:_____

_____

Location: _____

Appraisal: _____yes _____ no

Where kept? _____

To be given to whom: _____

Description: _____

_____

Location: _____

Appraisal: _____yes _____ no

Where kept? _____

To be given to whom: _____

Description: _____

_____

Location: _____

Appraisal: _____yes _____ no

Where kept? _____

To be given to whom: _____

Aftercare Information

Funeral Arrangements/Special Instructions

Mortuary: _____

Name:_____

Contact: _____

Address:_____

_____

Phone: _____

Fax: _____

Email: _____

Cemetery

Name:_____

Contact: _____

Address:_____

_____

Phone: _____

Fax: _____

Email: _____

Cemetery Plot Information: Location of Document

Special Funeral Instructions or Requests:

Letters

Upon the passing of a loved one, you will be responsible for communicating with companies, financial institutions, and any business that the senior dealt with. As challenging as this is for you, you can prepare in advance for this task and do it when you are ready. You will need numerous original copies of the death certificate (ten at a minimum and, depending upon the size of the estate or investments, you might need up to thirty). It is easier and more financially feasible to order these from the mortuary at the time of death. Security is heightened today and most companies require an original death certificate. You will need a death certificate to accompany most correspondence with businesses that you send letters of notification. It is almost impossible to cancel credit cards, telephone or cable service, insurance, vehicle loans, etc., over the phone. Be prepared to create a general letter that can be customized for each company you wish to alert. Generally speaking, the mortuary will communicate with Social Security and any government agencies.

Some of the people and places where letters may be needed:

- Attorney
- Accountant/Tax Advisor/Financial Planner
- Executor/Trustee
- Employer (if there is one or if a pension is involved)
- Veteran's Administration
- Insurance Companies
- Bank/Savings & Loan/Credit Union
- Medical/Dental Insurance
- Newspaper Delivery

- Leased Vehicles
- Finance/Loan Company
- Mortgage Loan Company
- Installment Loans
- Credit Card Companies
- Umbrella Liability Policy
- Homeowner's Insurance
- Landlord (if property is leased)
- Manager of Investment Property
- Tenants
- Utility Companies
- Phone Company/Internet/Cell Phone Provider
- Cable
- Veterinarian
- Doctors/Dentist
- Pharmacy
- Hospital
- Security Company
- Cancellation of Driver's License
- Gardener
- Pool Service
- Charitable Organizations
- Alumni, Clubs, or Social Organizations
- Memberships
- Magazine Subscriptions

Many of the above groups or businesses can be contacted by phone. If a letter is required, you will be told at the time of the call. Be gentle with yourself when taking on this task. This is a great time to ask for help from your support team or just friends who have reached out to you. You will be amazed at the outpouring of kindness from family and friends.

Afterword

Caregivers must have a quick learning curve and you will soon realize that having humility and asking for assistance are the only ways to survive without losing your mind. There is never enough time in the day for yourself and, if you have a family, it seems as though there is never enough time for them. At the end of the day, you climb into bed exhausted. In spite of the exhaustion, I was always filled with a sense of purpose because of making the human connection with a man who, for years, was just my ex-husband's father.

Little did I know that our relationship and friendship would enhance my life in ways I couldn't begin to imagine at the time. He passed away in July 2009 on a clear California morning. I was there when he left this world. In the end, we were so close that we had the ability to communicate in silence, but with complete understanding. A day doesn't pass that I don't think about him and miss him, but I am blessed for having known him.

Caregiving is vital and, if you are in the midst of it, know that you are making a difference, that you will get beyond it, that your life will be changed because of it, and that what you are doing matters; and isn't that what we are all really supposed to be doing in our time here?

"Caregiving is Soul Giving."

For Your Consideration

1. Consider joining a caregiver support group. Spending time once a week with people experiencing the same journey as you are is not only comforting, but allows an opportunity to learn from others. Most caregivers have solved problems in unique ways and they are happy to share their knowledge. It's also a great place to receive emotional support.

2. If you are suffering from caregiver burnout and you can't find your way out of it, you must get some professional help. See your doctor and ask for a referral. Your health and wellbeing are of the utmost importance.

3. Buy Long-Term Care Insurance. It may be too late to buy this insurance for your loved one, but it's not too late for you. Long-Term Care Insurance helps offset the caregiving costs and will make it possible for you to hire outside help. I can't stress this enough. Plan ahead.

4. Check out Adult Daycare Centers. There are wonderful centers all over the country for healthy, vital seniors. These centers give the senior specific activities to do during the day, help them socialize with others and helps stave off boredom and even depression.

5. Utilize as many public and non-profit services as you can. You do not need to do this alone.

6. Contact the local college or university and see if they have a gerontology or nursing program. This is a great resource for finding affordable help. Many students need credit and I encourage you to check this out.

7. If you notice your senior loved one acting out, behaving inappropriately, experiencing unnecessary anger or rage, do not assume that it's part of the aging process. Seek help immediately and have your loved one tested.

8. If you have children, try to get them involved. Children bring joy to the aging process. They do not need to be sheltered from an aging loved one in need of care. Involve them. We are one of the few societies which does not honor our elders. Maybe it's time to start thinking differently about this.

9. Keep a journal. At the end of the day, you are exhausted, but I can tell that by putting your thoughts and feelings on paper, you will free your mind and have a more restful sleep. In addition, journaling helps us express our deepest feelings, thoughts and ideas.

10. Keep your perspective and maintain a sense of humor. You will not live as a caregiver for the rest of your life. Celebrate the moments. Find humor in the journey.

11. Utilize your support team. Finding the right doctors is important. Making sure the house is safe is absolutely

necessary. Caring for yourself and not getting lost in the process is also your responsibility. Stop living in guilt and value yourself.

Recommended Reading

Chicken Soup for the Caregiver's Soul: Stories to Inspire Caregivers in the Home, the Community and the World (Chicken Soup for the Soul), by Jack Canfield, Mark Victor Hansen, LeAnn Thieman L.P.N., and Rosalynn Carter, Health Communications, Inc., 2004.

Making Rounds with Oscar: The Extraordinary Gift of an Ordinary Cat, David Dosa, M.D., Hyperion, 2010.

Elder Rage or Take My Father Please: How to Survive Caring For Aging Parents, Jacqueline Marcell, Impressive Press, 2001.

Emotional Renewal: Guided Imagery for Caregivers, Looking After Yourself While Helping a Loved One, Lynn Joseph, Ph.D., (DVD), Discovery Dynamics, Inc. 2008.

The Myth of Alzheimer's: What You Aren't Told About Today's Most Dreaded Diagnosis, Peter J. Whitehouse, St. Martin's Griffin, 2008.

Mental Housecleaning, Tomas Lafayette Picard. DC, Mental Housecleaning, LLC, 2009.

Take Your Oxygen First, Leeza Gibbons, James Huysman, PSYD, LCSW, Rosemary DeAnglelis Laird, M.D., LaChance Publishing, 2009.

Why Not Start Living Your Life Today, Eric Delabarre, Seven Publishing, 2003.

Resource Guide

60 Plus Association
www.60plus.org
1-703-560-7587
The 60 Plus Association is a non-partisan seniors advocacy group with a free enterprise, less government, less taxes approach to seniors issues. 60 Plus aims to end federal estate tax and ensuring Social Security for the next generation.

AARP
www.aarp.org
888-687-2277

Association of Mature American Citizens
www.amac.us
1-888-262-2006
An alternative to AARP

Aging Care
www.agingcare.com
A popular website created for families caring for aging loved ones. It offers advice, community and professionals who answer your questions on line. (Full disclosure: I am on their Board of Experts.)

Alzheimer's Disease and Related Disorders Association
www.ALZ.org
1-800-272-3900
The Alzheimer's Association is the leading voluntary health organization in Alzheimer care, support and research, which aims to eliminate Alzheimer's through research, as well as providing and expanding care and support for all those affected by the disease.

The Amen Clinic for Behavioral Medicine
www.brainplace.com
1-949-266-3700
Amen Clinics is dedicated to improving the lives of families through education, advancements in neuroimaging, and individualized treatment plans. They use the least toxic treatments for their patients, and use interventions from natural supplements, medications, dietary interventions, and targeted psychotherapy.

American Association of Geriatric Psychiatry
www.aagpgpa.org
1-301-654-7850
The Geriatric Mental Health Foundation raises awareness of psychiatric and mental health disorders, which affect the elderly, eliminate the stigma of having a mental illness, promote healthy aging techniques, and increase access to mental health care for the elderly.

American Cancer Society
www.cancer.org
1-866-228-4327
The American Cancer Society is the national, community-based, voluntary health organization that is dedicated to ending cancer as a major health problem by using preventive measures against cancer, saving lives, and ending suffering from cancer, through research, education, advocacy, and service. There are great links to having your own personal page on here with doctor's appointments and research that pertains to what is happening with your disease. Also there is a link about what is happening in your community and how to get involved.

American Health Care Association (Referrals to care facilities)
www.ahcancal.org
1-202-842-4444
AHCA represents the long-term care community of the nation to government, business leaders, and the general public. It also strives for change within the long-term care field, providing information, education, and administrative tools that enhance quality at every level.

American Psychiatric Association
www.PSYCH.org
1-202-682-6000

The APA is an organization composed primarily of medical specialists who are qualified psychiatrists or in the process of becoming qualified. There are over 38,000 member physicians who work together to ensure humane care and effective treatment for all persons with mental disorder.

American Seniors Association
www.AmericanSeniors.org
1-800-951-0017
The American Seniors Association's mission is to provide seniors with the choices, information, and services they need to live healthier, wealthier lives. The ASA prides itself on ensuring their members' dignity and security. It offers links to prescription discounts, Medicare solutions, insurance products, and even travel.

Arthritis Foundation
www.ARTHRITIS.org
The Arthritis Foundation is the only national non-profit organization that supports all different types of arthritis and related conditions. The foundation helps people affected by arthritis take control of the disease by providing public health education, pursuing public policy and legislation, and conducting evidence-based programs to improve the quality of life for those living with arthritis.

BenefitsCheckup
(A Service from the National Council on Aging)
www.benefitscheckup.org
BenefitsCheckUp is the nation's most comprehensive web-based service to screen for benefits programs for seniors with limited income and resources. It includes public and private benefits programs such as prescription drugs, nutrition, legal, healthcare, transportation, financial, and employment.

Children of Aging Parents
(Counseling and referrals to caregivers)
www.caps4caregivers.org
1-800-227-7294
Children of Aging Parents gives caregivers reliable information and advice through support groups, workshops, and presentations for churches, schools, employers, service clubs, and television audiences.

Comfort Keepers
www.comfortkeepers.com
1-800-387-2414
Comfort Keepers helps people live full, independent and dignified lives within the comfort of their own homes. Comfort Keepers is dedicated to providing in-home care that betters their clients' lives and helps them maintain the highest possible level of independent living. Comfort Keepers provides companionship, meal preparation, transportation, and light housework.

Eldercare Locator
www.eldercare.gov
1-800-677-1116
Eldercare Locator helps find local agencies in every state and community that can help the elderly and their families find home and community-based services like transportation, meals, home care, and caregiver services.

Eldercare Web
www.elderweb.com
1-309-451-3319
Eldercare Web offers a variety of links and information for caregivers, providers, and advisors to the elderly. The links include: advance directives, care facilities, financial plan fraud, abuse home care, nursing homes, and prescription costs.

★ **Elder Proofing the Home**
www.elderproofhome.com
The one company I truly trust to offer wise council, great products and services and they are efficient with reasonable pricing.

Family Caregiver
www.caregiver.org
1-800-445-8106
The FCA is a public voice for caregivers, which illustrates the daily challenges they face, offering them the assistance they so desperately need and deserve, and advocating their cause through education, services, and research.

firstSTREET
www.firststreetonline.com
firstStreet offers solutions for baby-boomers and seniors in the bedroom, bathroom, and kitchen, as well as, aids for vision and hearing. This website has products for the problems you face daily in your home.

Good Old Days Magazine
www.goodolddaysonline.com
1-800-829-5865
Good Old Days brings the nostalgic delight of stories, articles and pictures from bygone times.

HealingWell.com
www.healingwell.com
HealingWell.com is a community and information website for patients, caregivers, and families coping with diseases, disorders and chronic illness.

Hospice Foundation of America
www.hospicefoundation.org
1-800-854-3402
Hospice Foundation of America is a great website for those who personally or professionally cope with terminal illness and hospice care. It offers links to locate hospices near you, offers council for grief and loss, and also has a "caregiver corner." A nice feature of the website is that you change the font size, so it is easier to read!

Identity Theft—Federal Trade Commission
www.ftc.gov
Under the box "Quick Finder" on the homepage click on "identity theft." Good links are under the "Consumers" tab.

Long Term Care Living
www.LongTermCareLiving.com
This website offers a variety of features including a section that assess the loved one's needs in a long-term care facility. It also has a section devoted to advice for families, tips for making the move to a long-term care facility smooth, and information on how to pay for long-term care.

Macular Degeneration Partnership

www.AMD.org

1-310-623-4466

Macular Degeneration Partnership is a website that offers information online with helpful tips, a toolkit that you can request, as well as, sign up for an e-newsletter which gives update research and treatment for AMD.

Meals on Wheels Association of America

www.mowaa.org

Meals on Wheels is an organization that brings food to persons who are homebound.

Medical Alert

www.medicalalert.com

1-888-633-4298

Medical Alert is a service that provides medical identification bracelets and necklaces, and different types of membership benefits to choose from.

Medicare

www.medicare.gov

1-800-633-4227

The official link to the United States Government website of people with Medicare. There are links to information regarding billing, health records, plans, eligibility, and much more.

National Alliance for Caregiving

www.caregiving.org

The National Alliance for Caregiving is dedicated to providing support to family caregivers and the professionals who help them, as well as increasing public awareness of issues facing family caregivers.

National Association of Area Agencies on Aging

www.n4a.org

1-800-510-2020

n4a advocates on behalf its member agencies for services and resources for older adults and persons with disabilities. They work with their members to achieve a society that values and supports people as they age.

National Association for Home Care
www.nahc.org
1-202-547-7424
NAHC is the nation's largest trade association representing the interests and concerns of home care agencies, hospices, home care aide organizations, and medical equipment suppliers.

National Association of Professional Geriatric Care Managers
www.caremanager.org
1-520-881-8008
The NAGCM website has links to helping find a local care manager, information about what care managing is, important questions to ask when you are looking for a care manager, and many other helpful services for those and their families who are thinking of using a care manager in their life.

National Cancer Institute
www.nci.nih.gov
1-800-4-CANCER
The National Cancer Institute offers information about all different types of cancer, lists of clinical trials, and answers to commonly asked questions. This is a great website to begin with, if you have any questions about cancer.

National Association of Professional Organizers
www.napo.net
1-856-380-6828
The National Association of Professional Organizers (NAPO) is a group of about 4,200 professional organizers dedicated to helping individuals and businesses bring order and efficiency to their lives.

National Council on Aging
www.ncoa.org
1-202-479-1200
NCOA is private, nonprofit organization that provides information, training, technical assistance, advocacy, and leadership in all aspects of aging services and issues.

National Hospice and Palliative Care Organization
www.nhpco.org
1-703-837-1500
The NHPCO is the largest nonprofit membership organization representing hospice and palliative care programs and professionals in the United States. The organization is committed to improving end-of-life care and expanding access to hospice care with the goal of profoundly enhancing quality of life for people dying in America and their loved ones.

National Eye Institute
www.nei.nih.gov
National Eye Institute's mission is to "conduct and support research, training, health information dissemination, and other programs with respect to blinding eye diseases, visual disorders, mechanisms of visual function, preservation of sight, and the special health problems and requirements of the blind."

National Family Caregivers Association
www.nfcacares.org
1-301-942-6430
The National Family Caregivers Association educates, supports, empowers, and speaks up for Americans who care for loved ones with a chronic illness, disability, or the frailties of old age.

National Library of Medicine
www.medlineplus.gov
Medline Plus offers online information from the National Institute of Health including health topics, encyclopedia, drug information, and clinical trials.

National Mental Health Association
www.nmha.org
1-703-684-7722_
1-800-969-6642
The National Mental Health Association offers information on different health matters; where you can receive treatment; information about insurance, and answers to common questions.

National Osteoporosis Foundation

www.nof.org

Offers all information needed regarding osteoporosis and the questions that come with it.

National Parkinson Foundation

www.parkinson.org

Offers all information needed regarding Parkinson's disease and the questions that come with it. There is also information on how to adapt your lifestyle.

National Senior Citizens Education and Research Center

www.nscerc.org

1-301-578-8800

The NSCERC has information about senior living, retirement planning, nursing, asset management, and day-to-day care.

National Senior Citizens Law Center

www.nsclc.org

(202) 289-6976

The National Senior Citizens Law Center advocates before the courts, Congress and federal agencies to promote the independence and well-being of low-income elderly and disabled Americans.

Nursing Home Reports

www.freenursinghomereports.com

This website offers first account reviews of nursing homes, report cards from certain states, and nursing home ratings from federal inspections.

Retirement Research Foundation

www.rrf.org

1-773-714-8080

The Retirement Research Foundation is devoted to improving quality of life for the nation's older population by improving conditions for those who are vulnerable due to frailty associated with advanced age, those who are economically disadvantaged and at greatest risk of falling through the safety net, and those who experience disparities related to race and ethnicity.

Senior Corps
www.seniorcorps.com
1-800-424-8867
Senior Corps connects persons over fifty-five with the people and organizations that need them most. Senior Corps helps them become mentors, coaches or companions to people in need, or contribute their job skills and expertise to community projects and organizations.

Senior Housing Net
www.seniorhousingnet.com
Senior Housing Net offers links to types of housing and care, payment options, and moving and storage information. There are also helpful tips for making the loved senior citizen fill at home in their new living facility.

Senior Options
www.senioroptions.com
Senior Options is a nationwide guide to senior services such as long term care, eldercare locator, family caregiver, recreation centers, and retirement homes.

Social Security Administration
www.ssa.gov
The official Social Security Administration website.

Social Security Administration
www.ssa.gov/retire2
The official Social Security Administration website with a retirement planner.

Veterans Financial, Inc.
www.veteransfinancial.com
1-800-835-1541
Veterans Financial is a national company with a single purpose: to provide sound financial advice to older veterans and their families who may now or in the future need assistance either in an assisted living community, a nursing home setting, or in their own home.

Visiting Angels
www.visitingangels.com
1-800-365-4189
A leading, nationally respected network of non-medical, private duty home-care agencies providing senior care, elder care, personal care, respite care and companion care to help the elderly and adults continue to live in their homes across America.

Well Spouse Foundation
www.wellspouse.org
1-800-838-0879
The Well Spouse Foundation is a home for the husbands, wives and partners of those with any chronic illness, disease or disability. Well Spouse hopes you will find the information presented on their web site easy to navigate and helpful in your caregiver journey.

Write a Senior Citizen
www.writeseniors.com
Write a Senior Citizen is a great website that allows senior citizens to interact with people outside of their age group. There are lists of senior citizens who you can email and start a pen-pal friendship with.

Glossary

Activities of Daily Living (ADL). Daily activities such as personal grooming, cooking, eating, toileting, dressing, doing laundry, etc.

Advance directives. Legal documents expressing a person's wishes should he/she become unable to make medical, legal, or personal decisions.

Adverse drug reaction. A harmful or unpleasant reaction from a medication or the result of two or more drugs reacting negatively with each other.

Aging in place. The ability of an individual to remain in one's own home or current residence as long as possible.

Alzheimer's disease. A form of dementia; an irreversible, degenerative brain disorder that causes progressive loss of memory and cognitive function.

Assessment. An evaluation of an individual's physical, psychological, emotional, social, and environmental needs, usually performed by a registered nurse or social worker.

Apnea. A temporary suspension of breathing. (Sleep apnea is a disorder where breathing can slow down or stop during sleep.)

Assisted devices. Any type of equipment that aids an individual, such as a walker, wheelchair, reachers, hand rails, etc.

Bedsore. A pressure-induced ulceration of the skin and subcutaneous tissue caused by poor circulation and prolonged pressure on body parts, esp. bony protuberances, often occurs in bedridden or immobile patients. Also called *decubitus ulcer, pressure sore*. (Check the body frequently for signs of breakdown of the skin.)

Caregiver. Any individual who provides personal, emotional, financial, or supportive care for another person. A caregiver can be a paid professional or a volunteer.

Certified Nursing Assistant (CAN). A person who earns a state license or certification by completing specific homecare and patient training.

Chronic Obstructive Pulmonary Disease (COPD). Any of a variety of lung diseases leading to poor pulmonary aeration (supply the blood with oxygen), including emphysema and chronic bronchitis.

Cognitive impairment. A decline in one's ability to perform tasks, think clearly, or make decisions. (This is one of the first signs that something is wrong or has changed and you need to pay attention to it.)

Compliance. The ability to respond appropriately to another person's directions. For example: complying with a physician's orders or complying with dietary restrictions.

Congestive Heart Failure (CHF). A condition in which the heart fails to pump adequate amounts of blood to the tissues, resulting in an accumulation of blood returning to the heart from the veins. This is often accompanied by distension of the ventricles, edema, and/or shortness of breath.

Decubitus ulcer. See bedsore.

Dementia. Severe impairment or loss of intellectual capacity resulting in memory loss, personality changes, language problems, mood swings, and an inability to learn or retain information.

Diabetes. Disease caused by any or all of several metabolic disorders and often marked by excessive discharge of urine. Some of the signs in the elderly are persistent thirst and open sores that will not heal.

Do Not Resusitate (DNR). Part of an advanced medical directive, a legal document order to not resuscitate an individual whose heart or breathing stops. Specifics vary by state.

Edema. An excessive amount of watery fluid accumulating in cells, tissues, or body cavities. Edema can be mild and benign—often occurs after prolonged standing in the elderly; or a serious sign of pulmonary, heart, liver, or kidney failure, or other diseases.

Heart attack. Damage to a heart muscle due to loss of blood supply, often caused by blockage of a coronary artery, symptoms vary widely and can include chest discomfort or pain, upper body pain, stomach pain, shortness of breath, anxiety, lightheadedness, sweating, and nausea/vomiting. (Women and the elderly often have atypical or more subtle symptoms.)

Heart disease. An abnormality of the heart, or of the blood vessels supplying the heart, that impairs normal function.

High Blood Pressure (HBP). Elevation of the arterial blood pressure or a condition resulting from it; hypertension. Chronic high blood pressure is dangerous and should be monitored regularly.

Hospice care. A concept of care, not a place. Hospice care is a team approach to caregiving, and involves nurses, social workers, home health aides, and even chaplains, to administer care to patients and their families. When an individual has a life-limiting illness (usually no more than six months to live) they are often referred to hospice.

Incontinence. Inability to restrain natural discharges or evacuations of urine or feces. (Many elderly persons are placed in a nursing home when this happens. Use undergarments.)

Licensed Vocational Nurse (LVN). A licensed practical nurse authorized by license to practice in California or Texas.

Low Blood Pressure (LBP). Decreased or lowered blood pressure (also called hypotension.) Chronic low blood pressure is dangerous and should be monitored regularly.

Medicaid. A federal program mandated by individual states to provide coverage for certain medical care costs. The program assists individuals with a limited income. Covers some care at home and/or in a nursing home.

Medicare. A federal program for individuals age sixty-five and older. Benefit areas are divided into three parts: Part A—hospital benefits; Part B—medical benefits; Part C—Medicare + Choice.

Medigap. Private supplemental insurance plan designed to cover some of the costs not covered by Medicare or only partially covered by Medicare.

Palliative care. A specialized care focused on the pain, symptoms, and stress of serious illness. (If possible, find a hospital or medical center in your area that has a palliative care program. Palliative care is not the same as hospice care.)

Patient advocate. Usually a registered nurse, social worker, or volunteer who acts on behalf of the patient as an intermediary between the patient and the medical team or hospital.

Personal care attendant (PCA).A person who assists an individual with a disability or other health care needs in activities of daily living, such as bathing, dressing, housecleaning, meal preparation, feeding, etc.

Podatrist. A doctor specialized in the care of the foot, ankle, and lower leg. Chronic foot problems occur in the elderly for a variety of reasons. Reduced flexibility makes toenail and foot care difficult. Toenails need attention. Schedule a regular appointment with a podiatrist for proper foot care. Watch for small open cuts on feet that do not heal (a possible sign of diabetes). Trim nails regularly and keep feet clean and moisturized. Be on the alert for purplish-colored feet as this is a sign of poor circulation.

PRN. Direction of schedule for taking of prescription medications as needed.

Registered nurse (RN). A graduate trained nurse who has been licensed by a state authority after passing qualifying examinations for registration.

Respite care or respite services. Care provided on a temporary basis to relieve the ongoing duties and stress of a caregiver.

Stroke. A sudden loss of brain function caused by a blockage or rupture of a blood vessel to the brain. It is often characterized by loss of muscular control, reduced level of or loss of sensation or consciousness, dizziness, slurred speech, paralysis (often on the left side of the body) or other symptoms that vary with the extent and severity of the damage to the brain.

Urinary tract infection (UTI). A bacterial infection occurring anywhere in the urinary tract. (The elderly are extremely susceptible to UTIs usually due to poor bladder emptying and incontinence and their compromised immune system.)

About the Author

Cindy Laverty discovered that compassionate caregiving was her true calling several years ago while caring for Bob, her aging and former father-in-law. She is the Founder of The Care Company, which is dedicated to resolving the multitude of issues which face seniors and families. She is the host of The Cindy Laverty Show, a weekly, commercial radio program dedicated to Cindy's philosophy that we need to learn how to care for ourselves so we can better care for each other.

In addition, Cindy is a speaker, conducts seminars to help others with the caregiving journey and she does one-on-one coaching for caregivers seeking personal help and support. Cindy is there for you each step of the way and she is "The Compassionate Caregiver's Best Friend."™

You can contact Cindy or learn more about The Care Company by visiting her websites:

www.thecarecompany.biz

www.cindylavertyshow.com

NOTES

NOTES